TOTAL
POTENTIAL

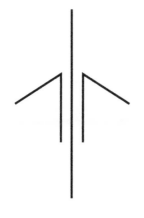

TOTAL POTENTIAL

HOW TO CREATE A CULTURE OF GROWTH
AND WELLNESS SO YOUR WHOLE FAMILY CAN THRIVE

COLE BERSCHBACK
& JAKE TAYLOR

thetotalpotential.com

Published and distributed by Merack Publishing.

Library of Congress Control Number: 2021916331
Berschback, Cole and Taylor, Jake
Total Potential: How to Create a Culture of Growth and Wellness So Your Whole Family Can Thrive

Paperback ISBN 978-1-949635-76-8
Hardcover ISBN 978-1-949635-78-2
eBook ISBN 978-1-949635-77-5

DEDICATION

For our families:
Haley, Jax, and Dylan
John, Andrew, Will and Taylor

CONTENTS

INTRODUCTION

Wait a minute! I spend my days running, trying to be my best as a spouse, parent, friend, coworker, community member, and world citizen. Yet, I'm running on fumes, not able to give my best to anyone as I sprint toward some imaginary finish line. My self-help books tell me to do this on my own, but where do my partner and children fit into all of this? We wondered the same thing. This book will teach you how to cultivate your best self within the context of your family, to create a culture of growth and wellness in which your whole family can thrive! We call this a journey of mastery—a journey of always becoming more while being content in the process. It begins with personal development. The concepts and tools that help us become our best as an individual also apply to our marriage and family. We can become happier and healthier in our marriage and more connected as a family.

We have been taught to be constantly chasing—CEO status, wealth, a large house with a five-car garage, successful kids who achieve straight A's and go on to play college sports. But we get those things and what happens? Nothing. We are still the same human. And that human wakes up the day after crossing that imaginary finish line of success with exactly the same character, emotions, body, thoughts, and needs. There is only one finish line we are going to cross in this life – the one just before our obituary is written. Instead of chasing things, let's chase our character, our development, our connections. The things that allow every day to be filled with joy, peace, love. Life isn't what happens once we own our dream house.

Life is what happens in the meantime.

As Archbishop Desmond Tutu said in The Book of Joy, "We are all masterpieces in the making" (Gyatso and Tutu 2016, 92). Becoming a masterpiece is the process of our life. We are always becoming more. We just have to decide what we want to become.

HOW WILL THIS BOOK HELP ME?

Is it time to break the cycle of living unconsciously? We are going to offer tools to help you and your family live a purpose-filled, growth-oriented life. We want to help you become aware of the little moments and enjoy the daily process of family life—not numbly go through the motions. Not basing your happiness on some far-off result.

We'll explore how you and your family can build and maintain strong physical bodies, doing so in ways that can be fun together. We'll learn how to develop discipline to stay the course and a mindset that is positive and balanced. Finally, we will reach inside and work on developing our spiritual realm. We'll discover ways to connect with our inner being, our higher power, and with those we care about. Contentment is the culmination of the spiritual realm. We will learn how to be content on our journey and embrace discomfort as a learning opportunity.

You can start wherever you currently are on your life journey. You may find that you are advanced in some areas and need more help in other areas. That is completely normal. This book is meant to be a learning tool as well as a means of self-reflection. Grab a journal. You're going to want to take notes and use the prompts to flush out your biggest opportunities for tapping into your total potential

WHY WE WROTE THIS BOOK

We wrote this book as a brother-sister team. Like many authors who feel compelled to write about their enlightening experiences, we both hit the proverbial rock bottom—a dark, murky place.

I, Cole, survived a head-on collision with a drunk driver when I was nineteen years old. Defying the odds, somehow, I lived. While I spent months recovering, I kept coming back to the thought, The only reason I survived that accident is because of love—the love of my family and the love of my Higher Power. My family continues to be my sacred space. My husband and three children are my sanctuary. I have a drive to help others find their sacred space within their families as well.

My trials may be surprising to some people. I, Jake, was a professional hockey player, growing up with tunnel vision and a sole focus on hockey. Yes, my ego was stroked because I made it to the pro's; however, the only self-worth I had was tied to hockey. Even that wasn't consistent. If I wasn't performing well or pleasing everyone, my self-worth plunged. I didn't have a clue what self-reflection and empathy were or how they could benefit me. I was used to hearing coaches yell, "Crush them!" and "Work harder, you lazy oafs!" Internally, I was living a life full of anger and negativity mixed with an unhealthy dose of anxiety. I rationalized those feelings, though, because they made me play better and more aggressively on the ice. Then, I retired. That's when the bottom slid out from underneath me. I didn't know how to do life, how to find the real, authentic Jake. Through work, determination, my faith, and the love of my family, I have found home—inside myself. Now I'm able to give to others, including my wife and two children.

As we searched for resources to get healthy and lead more purposeful lives, we both found that one crucial component was missing—the inclusion of our families. One coach said we should exercise three hours at the gym every day to get healthy, but doing so would mean three more hours away from our families. Another source said we should meal-prep every meal, yet we knew our kids would never eat those meals. A yoga guru suggested this work is only possible when we live more like a solitary monk, that our family members were obstacles to enlightenment. Our family as obstacles? Everything that we heard and read encouraged us to pull away from our family and focus solely on ourselves.

Too often, we witnessed struggle amongst our married friends when one of the two tried to get healthy. One partner would embark on a profound journey of self-improvement—a yoga path, an extreme diet, a punishing exercise regimen. Their spouse was left in the dust, wondering what the hell just happened. Spouse tried to lasso the Enlightened Partner, to pull them and their new way of living back to what felt normal and comfortable. Consequently, the Enlightened Partner felt stifled and sabotaged. Instead of making their lives better, the self-improvement changes shattered family relationships. Hours were spent away from family, hours at the gym meant hours with a new guy, and family dinners couldn't be had in accordance with the new extreme diet limits. Ultimately a number of divorces occurred.

What happens when we try to become physically, mentally, and spiritually healthy, yet the rest of our family continues their old habits? The kids continue to come home from school, say a quick, clipped "Hello!", then flop into a chair to watch TV. All while maintaining a diet of chips, processed food, and orange soda. It is hard to sustain healthy practices when those around us don't understand or support our changes, changes interpreted as "ruining their lives!" We humans naturally don't like change. We are most comfortable maintaining the status quo. Lifestyle modifications can create growing rifts among family members.

But we don't want this for ourselves or our families. We want to develop deep, authentic relationships. We both knew from a young age that we someday wanted a family. We went through the excitement of planning and growing our families. Now that we have school-aged children, the norm seems to be to complain about our families. "I have to drive my kids from Chicago to New York this weekend for soccer!" and "My kids are driving me crazy! They are slobs. I spend most of my time cleaning up after them!" But wait! Didn't we want families? Aren't our families our most precious commodities?

We realized that we don't want to be the norm. We want to be uncommon. We want to be weird! We love our family and want to develop our greatest potential together, both as individuals and as a team.

In this book, we share our expertise in the areas of physical wellness and nutrition. We also share our experiences and hard-earned lessons from navigating personal wellness, marriage, and family life. Though neither of us is a psychologist or neuroscientist, we are educated and are self-professed learning junkies.

Cole is a registered dietitian and certified yoga instructor. She has spent her career helping others find their best through physical wellness. Now, as a certified Unbeatable Mind coach, she enjoys helping others connect to their emotional and spiritual selves, to master themselves to powerfully serve others.

Jake is a retired professional hockey player with seven seasons in the American Hockey League. Currently, in addition to his day job as Director of Sports Management at a wealth management firm, he is a CrossFit Level 1 trainer, Unbeatable

Mind coach, and hockey coach. He loves to regularly push his physical limits.

We are also normal, everyday lab rats who found the impetus to make a change. We continue to experiment on ourselves to see what works and what doesn't work as we travel on our journeys. We have learned to love the process, the joys, and the discomforts. This book is about making small adjustments every day. There is no one correct answer for everyone. Through practice and contemplation, you will find what works for you and your family.

Ideally, you and your partner will both read this book. The subject is about you, the relationship with your partner, and the relationships with your children. A number of ideas, practices, and contemplation exercises involve the participation of your partner and children—it's about realizing your total potential together! Consider using this book as a workbook, a learning tool. Each family member will benefit from having their own journal before embarking on this journey. When we transmit our thoughts to writing, we often discover some hidden gems lurking in our brains. Writing also helps commit new concepts to memory. Your children may even opt to draw ideas or feelings in their journals. Wonderful! As long as you are willing to continually learn and grow throughout your journey, this book will serve you.

BUILDING OUR STRONG HOME

We need to have a strong self before we can effectively give to others. A capable body, a clear mind, and a compassionate spirit will produce an abundant supply of energy, energy needed to help ourselves and our loved ones grow and thrive. We will use the idea of building and maintaining a home as an analogy to building and maintaining our self. In this book, we are going to build a mind-blowing, amazing home. We are going to name our home—The Self. It will be a place of profound joy and peace. It is going to be a safe, comfortable place while being strong enough to weather all types of storms. This is our forever home. The unique aspect of this home is that its construction will never end. We will continue building The Self until we die.

Each part is equally important. As you will see, they have different functions, and they have the potential to integrate seamlessly with one another.

- The Body consists of the foundation and framing of our home.

- The Mind is the internal wiring, the brains of our home.

- The Spirit is the flow of energy in our home.

Before we begin building The Self, we need to become familiar with the tools we are going to use. Seven power tools. We will use all seven when working on each section of The Self. We will describe them and provide opportunities to practice them as we start construction. Our power tools consist of courage, simplicity, positivity, commitment, resilience, awareness, and purpose. Some of the power tools have functions that overlap and need to be used together to work best.

While construction of The Self is ongoing, and though we can toggle between the various parts of The Self while relating to our power tools, we describe the journey in three steps:

1) The foundation and framing—Body

   a. Strong but flexible supports—Movement

   b. High-quality materials—Nutrition

2) The internal wiring, the brains—Mind

   a. Consistent actions that include a backup plan—Discipline

   b. Stable functioning but modifiable for change—Mindset

3) The flow of energy throughout the house—Spirit

   a. Room design for self-reflection and for gathering with loved ones—Connection

   b. Favorite chair in front of the fireplace during the life-long construction project—Contentment

Just like with a home, it makes sense to begin construction with the foundation and framing. This needs to be strong to support all other aspects of the home. We will use Movement to build strength and resilience in our Body. Our foundation and framing also need high-quality materials for strength and endurance. Nutrition will be our Body's high-quality materials.

Once our framing is up, we will work on the house's internal conduits. The internal wiring makes up the brains of the home.

The wiring needs to be consistent and function according to plans. We will learn to use Discipline to follow an action plan in the Mind chapter. The wiring needs to be stable yet able to be modified for inevitable future changes. We will learn about Mindset to examine our long-held, stable beliefs while challenging ourselves to keep expanding our minds.

Finally, we get to the most intimate and personal part of our home. We will create our rooms. We will design large gathering spaces to connect with our loved ones. To connect with our inner selves, we will create some small, quiet rooms. In the Spirit chapter, we will discuss why and how to create deep Connections with our authentic selves, our loved ones, and the Divine. Some of these connections will become so beautiful that they will bring us to tears. Lastly, while the preceding home construction continues to occur, we will place our favorite, comfortable chair next to the fireplace. In our Spirit self, this is contentment. It is inner peace, our safe haven regardless of what is going on around us.

Again, we'll never be done building The Self. It will always be a masterpiece in the making.

CHARACTER POWER TOOLS

We shape our tools,
and afterward our tools shape us.
— Marshall McLuhan

Through research, experience, and examining traditions from the east to the west, we have found seven power tools that are most effective at building a solid, strong Self. These tools have functions that overlap and correspond with one another. Unfortunately, we don't own the tools—yet. We have to practice using them in order to earn them.

Courage, Simplicity, Positivity, Commitment, Resilience, Awareness, and Purpose: the almighty power tools we will use to develop and refine all aspects of our Self. The power tools are also known by their slightly feebler term, "character traits."

However, are these traits a part of everyone's character? Only when we act on and align our behavior with them, do the traits become parts of our character. We need to practice them in order to claim them as our own.

We will eventually use the power tools so often that they will feel like an additional body part. The tools will become a part of us. We will own them. Instead of practicing courage, we will become courageous.

CHAPTER 1

COURAGE

**If one has courage, nothing can dim
the light that shines from within.
- Maya Angelou**

Courage is the first big move toward living a life that matters. Courage allows us to embrace life, be authentic, and eventually make decisions because we know what is truly important.

Courage is choosing to act despite our fears and discomfort, and despite the known and unknown risks. It can come in many forms—doing the right thing regardless of what people think, telling the truth, admitting when we are wrong or simply don't know the answer, venturing into the unknown, and ultimately being vulnerable. Courage is our choice to do something true yet is often uncomfortable.

We, as humans, naturally balk at discomfort. We even structure our lives in such a manner to avoid it. Discomfort is not intense pain. It is an uneasy feeling of being outside of our comfort zone. Our minds may fear the discomfort of starting a project, exercising, saying No, trying new activities, or sitting quietly to practice our breathing. What if we were to think of discomfort as a helpful signal? Rather than running from it or seeking distractions, what if we just sit with the feeling? Get curious about it. We will realize that the uncomfortable feeling will eventually go away. It is not permanent. What is the discomfort telling us? As we continue to practice sitting with feelings of discomfort, we will progressively develop a stronger sense of courage. In most cases, the fear of being uncomfortable is more painful than the actual situation we are afraid of in the first place.

COURAGE AND PERFECTIONISM

Not only do we humans dislike being uncomfortable, but we also don't like to fail. Similar to discomfort, some people are so afraid of failing that they simply avoid taking action. They don't even try. Others who fear failure may numb themselves with alcohol or drugs. Enter perfectionism—the fear of failure. Perfectionists subconsciously choose a tense life of fear over a more fulfilled life of opportunities. So why does it seem easier to succumb to fear? Look at our society. It is rather perfectionistic. Yes, companies exist in which failures are encouraged, but these do not represent the cultural norm. How do we try new things, grow, and improve without making mistakes, without failing? Even our school systems honor perfection—straight A's if a student's work is perfect, B's and C's if a student makes mistakes. It is not surprising that students fear failure in school. If they receive poor grades, they get punished—extracurricular activities get withheld, their colleges of choice are denied. Yet those who feel ruled by perfectionism are generally not joyful people; they are internally anxious. It is not fun to feel controlled by fear or the opinions of others. Perfectionists are typically not striving for excellence—they are trying to avoid failing or disappointing people. Researchers say that perfectionists are made, not born. This means that we can unlearn perfectionism and choose courage. We can decide to be brave.

COURAGE AND VULNERABILITY

Merriam-Webster defines vulnerability as "capable of being physically or emotionally wounded; open to attack or damage." Neither of these definitions makes us want to enroll in the next vulnerability class at the local community college. But doesn't this definition sound similar to the meaning of courage? Both require risk, and both potentially involve discomfort. Why on earth would we choose to be courageous and vulnerable? As the reigning queen of vulnerability, Brene Brown, said at the end of a Teddy Roosevelt quote,

> I want to be in the arena. I want to be brave with my life. And when we make the choice to dare greatly, we sign up to get our asses kicked. We can choose courage, or we can choose comfort, but we can't have both. Not at the same time. Vulnerability is not winning or losing; it's having the courage to show up and be seen when we have no control of the outcome. (Brown 2015, 267)

Men, even more so than women, have a long history of armoring up to avoid being vulnerable. From an early age, men are taught that vulnerability equals weakness. "Stop your crying," or "Don't show your emotions like a little girl!" To be truthful when afraid or uncomfortable, to cry, and to love without fear of rejection are not examples of weaknesses. They are signs of bravery. Vulnerability is actually a strength, a practice of courage. Courage and vulnerability allow us to be authentic, to live a life that is our own—one that we design— not a life other people have scripted for us. Courage allows us to experience life on a deeper and more meaningful level. It may leave us open to a few raised eyebrows or outright rejections from others, but so what? These risks pale in comparison to the potential of experiencing skin-tingling love, intimate relationships, and a hidden well of creativity.

As we move forward, think about making choices that are bold and uncomfortable. If you periodically decide to choose the easier way, don't think of it as a setback. We will be making small, daily tweaks in our lives. We'll start by practicing courage in small doses.

TIME FOR CONTEMPLATION

Contemplation involves creating time to specifically think about courage. Use any mode of reflection that is meaningful to you—prayer, meditation, breathing practice, yoga, walking in nature, etc. After reading the chapter about courage, what parts resonate with you?

IN YOUR JOURNAL, CONSIDER THE FOLLOWING QUESTIONS:

1. Give some examples of when I acted with courage. What conditions made it possible for me to act with courage?

2. In what ways have I limited myself when I've lacked courage?

3. In my marriage, when have I lacked the courage to love completely? What steps can I take now to start to turn this around?

4. How can I model courage for my children?

CHAPTER 2

SIMPLICITY

Possessions, outward success, publicity, luxury—to me
these have always been contemptible. I believe that
a simple and unassuming manner of life is best for
everyone, best for both the body and mind.
— Albert Einstein

When we think of the word simplicity, our minds may immediately go to the now-famous author and television personality, Marie Kondo. She is the modern guru of organizing and tidying up our home. Simplicity may apply to a purposefully organized home in which every toy, dish, and piece of mail has its designated resting place. But simplicity is more. It is about intentionally choosing the things in our life that are most meaningful, then focusing on them. The process then includes downsizing the remaining clutter, the not-so-important stuff, that distracts us from what we've deemed important.

Books, podcasts, and blogs offer a plethora of information about living more simply. We are not recommending that you sell your big house and SUV, set up a homestead off the grid, and grow your own food. Although more power to you if that is your thing! Choosing to live simply means choosing to apply our limited energy to what we've decided is most valuable to us. That, in turn, contributes to feelings of joy and fulfillment.

So, let's think about the average American life during this time in which we live. Do you think simplicity is a power tool that most people use? It almost seems like a badge of honor to describe how busy—how un-simple—our lives are. We don't even experience quality downtime anymore due to the 24/7 opportunity to be connected to our devices. As Josh Becker said, "We don't consider that, though devices connect us to the world, they disconnect us from ourselves" (Becker 2018, 22). They also disconnect us from our family. We are physically running around like hamsters on a spinning wheel while we are mentally playing Whack-a-Mole! We wonder why we are exhausted, crabby, envious, and apt to easily blame society for our busyness. It is time to hop off the wheel and plug up those mole holes. Let's resolve to focus on the aspects of our lives that bring us meaning.

Simplicity is often a significant mind shift for people. However, it does not mean laziness or lack of ambition. Simplified commitments may still be time-consuming, but they are specific ones that you've decided have meaning. They feed your soul.

SIMPLIFY TO UNCOVER YOUR PRIORITIES

Let's take time to assess the daily inputs and outputs associated with our lives.

1. In your journal—or a piece of scratch paper if you'd rather dispose of it—brainstorm everything that takes up your time. This may include childcare, errands, commutes to your children's school and practices, work outside the home, e-mail and other communications, social media, meal prep and meals themselves, house cleaning, homework help, dates with your spouse, etc.

2. Now consider the relationships that you keep. List them all, even those with whom you interact at your children's activities and athletic events.

3. Now only circle the things, commitments, and relationships that you absolutely love, that fill you up, that give your life meaning.

4. Without worrying about what anybody else will think, cross off anything on the list that feels unfulfilling, unconstructive, draining, or inauthentic.

This completed list is your first attempt at simplifying your life. Your circled items are your top priorities. Focus most of your energy on these. Your next priorities are those items on the list that you neither circled nor crossed out. Your last priorities are your crossed-out items. (Are they even priorities then?)

To help you focus on your priorities each day, consider doing a mini version of this exercise every morning.

POSITIVE ENERGY IS WAITING

Simplicity is associated with positive energy. When we decide to whittle down our lives, we reveal what truly gives our lives meaning. We put a limit on the negative forces that previously influenced our lives. Precious space will open up, allowing us to focus and live our lives with more purpose.

Choosing simplicity will be a powerful, rewarding change for you and your family. Your family has unknowingly risen to the top of your priority list—not that they weren't always right up there—because you consciously chose those relationships as ones that you treasure. Remember the shallow relationships, the ones that zap your energy because they are negative or judgmental? Did they remain on your edited priority list?

COMPLEXITY AND BOREDOM MAY SERVE A PURPOSE

Sometimes a complicated, complex life serves a need we aren't even aware of. Complexity is an effective distraction, a cover, a protection. Yet, underneath all of this, we may discover feelings of sadness, fear, or discontent. When our lives are simple, we have the time and space to address uncomfortable feelings. We don't feel such a need to layer up and protect ourselves with possessions and commitments.

Think back to a time when you were bored. Yes, you'll probably need to go back to your childhood. Our lives were simpler. What did you do when you were bored? Did you eventually get creative, use your imagination, invent magical worlds? Certain areas of our brain that foster creativity become activated when we are bored or under-stimulated. Psychologist Dr. Sandi Mann states that "When we are bored, we're searching for something to stimulate us that we can't find in our immediate surroundings. Once we start daydreaming and allow our minds to wander, we start thinking beyond our conscious" (Mann 2016). Artists, musicians, and writers consider boredom a gift, a gift that they can unwrap and release their creative ideas. Maybe we can do the same.

TIME FOR CONTEMPLATION

Create some time to specifically think about simplicity. Use any mode of reflection that is meaningful to you—prayer, meditation, breathing practice, yoga, walking in nature, etc. After reading the chapter about simplicity, what parts resonate with you?

IN YOUR JOURNAL, CONSIDER THE FOLLOWING QUESTIONS:

1. Is physical clutter an issue for our family? How does it distract us? What other types of clutter do we have? What are we ready to let go of?

2. Am I attached strictly to the things or the memories and people associated with those things?

3. How can I schedule boredom into my life?

4. In my marriage, how can we take time to simply focus on each other without distractions?

5. How can I model simplicity for my children?

CHAPTER 3

POSITIVITY

Watch your thoughts; they become words. Watch
your words; they become actions. Watch your
actions; they become habits. Watch your habits; they
become character. Watch your character; it becomes
your destiny.
— Lao Tzu

Positivity is a decision. Based on the above quote by Lao Tzu, a positive mindset can ultimately lead to a joyful life. People actually decide to have a positive outlook, to see the joy and possibilities in life. Some people seem to have a genetic propensity for positivity; it comes easily for them. For those of us who are more cynically inclined, we need to reframe our perspective.

It may sound Pollyanna-like to simply reframe our perspective from one that is negative or neutral to one that is positive.

Number one: It's not simple to reframe our perspective. It takes concentrated practice. It's actually easier and more natural to choose a negative focus. Our brains are evolutionarily wired for negativity. During the era of the saber-toothed tiger, negativity kept us alive.

Number two: Our brains need a ratio of five positive thoughts to one negative thought—just to create a neutral thought. So, reframing our perspective from a negative one to a positive one is not going to turn us into a Pollyanna, one who sees only rainbows and unicorns. We have to work the hell out of our positivity power tool to overcome the negative tendencies of our society and our brain.

To develop a positive perspective, we need to look for possibilities instead of dead ends. We need to alter our outlook from a can't do attitude to a can-do, realistic attitude. A positive perspective encourages our brain to look for options and figure out solutions. It expands our creative-thinking potential.

Reframing our perspective requires us to become aware of our thoughts. Once we pay attention to and identify our thoughts, we can begin to address them. You may have heard the term metacognition—thinking about our thinking. When fully developed, this higher-level function of our brain can assess the numerous thoughts that go through our minds. If we identify a negative thought, we can ask, "Is this thought true? Is it helping me right now?"

Dr. David Hawkins describes how positivity has been proven to have physical and psychological benefits. It changes our biochemistry. People who have a positive outlook live longer.

Positivity helps us make better decisions more quickly and be more productive. (Hawkins 2012) It propels us forward. Our relationships benefit since our behavior toward others improves. People want to be around positive people. This positivity tool almost sounds like a healthy recreational drug!

We can't talk about positivity without addressing the pervasive feelings of stress. Stress is tension that can be physical, mental and emotional. It contributes to nearly every medical ailment. It affects our sleep, our body habits, our ability to focus, and our relationships. Yet, we can control our stress. We minimize stress by addressing our thoughts, by reframing our perspective to one that is positive. We can even apply positivity to our memories. Before memories are laid down, our brain adds a spin on the events that just took place. Our brain applies a narrative to the facts. This creates a memory that has meaning and makes sense. In other words, our memories are stories. What if we changed the narrative to one that is positive?

IMPACT OF NEGATIVITY

Since we are touting the benefits of positivity, let's acknowledge the impact negativity has on our lives. When we have a negative perspective, it narrows our way of thinking. It shuts down our thought processes, so we blame and complain about why things don't work.

Let's take the example of the saber-toothed tiger. When our brave, agile ancestors came in contact with the saber-toothed tiger, their brains quickly registered fear. Fear physically prepared their bodies for a life-or-death situation. Fear continues to have the same effect on our body today as if we are being chased by the extinct feline. It is a normal, necessary emotion—but one that should only be short-lived.

Fear is a negative emotion. Anger, stress, and disgust are further examples of negative emotions. Yes, we need to feel these emotions. And we need to let them go. Negative emotions, when we hold onto them, can hurt us. We are still programmed to respond to negative emotions in the same way as our ancestors—by going into fight, flight, or freeze mode. We develop tunnel vision; we hyper-focus. We can't problem-solve. The rest of the world doesn't matter at that point. These reactions are simply not helpful today when, for example, an impatient driver passes and shows us his longest finger.

Positivity takes relentless practice. It takes work and focus. We need to be prepared to take a different route when negativity jumps into our path. Eventually, our positivity power tool will help us turn obstacles into opportunities along our journey.

TIME FOR CONTEMPLATION

Does it ever feel like negativity comes in cycles? When something we view as negative happens, we tend to look for other negative things. Mindfulness, meditation, yoga, and deep breathing—clearing our minds—can help stop the negative cycles. These practices promote a positive mindset. During your meditation on positivity, think about what you are grateful for. Think outside the box. Fresh blades of grass, fluffy clouds on a sunny day, your child's piano tunes, or even slapping a mosquito before it takes a bite?

Create time to specifically think about positivity. Use any mode of reflection that is meaningful to you—prayer, meditation, breathing practice, yoga, walking in nature, etc. After reading the chapter about positivity, what parts resonate with you?

IN YOUR JOURNAL, CONSIDER THE FOLLOWING QUESTIONS:

1. Name some things that bring me joy.

2. When I feel negative, what is happening within my body? Do I feel tension anywhere?

3. What am I grateful for in my partner? In what ways can I practice positivity with my partner?

4. Think of a situation that has been challenging for you. Visualize how you would ideally want to handle that situation. Without anger or frustration, what steps are you taking to resolve it? See it having a peaceful end. Write down the key factors that made this situation successful. You can come back to this as a reminder.

5. Where can I easily be more positive with my children?

6. What positive behaviors do my children have that I can help them grow, appreciate, or focus on?

7. How can I model positivity for my children?

CHAPTER 4

COMMITMENT

It takes deep commitment to change and an even
deeper commitment to grow.
— Ralph Ellison

Commitment is the decision to take that first, proverbial, single step. Our ultimate goal may seem far out of reach at this point. That is okay. We are a single step closer to it. We are moving toward meaningful change and growth. We can think of commitments as long-term vows or promises. But they are choices, not obligations or requirements. For commitments to be successful, they have to be related to a deep purpose—our own personal, meaningful reason why. What is the underlying reason we want to make this commitment? How will this commitment help us become better?

We are not talking about egocentric vows such as, "I am going to lose weight to stun the pants off my previous classmates at my high school reunion," or "I am going to beef up to scare the hell out of Ronnie, the kid who bullied me in middle school." The joy of hitting such results fades rather quickly. Our ego isn't satisfied for long. We don't sustain the effort needed to accomplish egocentric outcomes—once we've achieved our goal, we are done. These goals often consist of hitting numbers or checking boxes. They are often associated with stress and a sense of urgency.

So, how do we effectively honor our commitments?

PERSONAL COMMITMENTS VERSUS FAMILY COMMITMENTS

Commitment is a mindset. When we are committed to something, we've decided it has meaning. Personal commitments have long-term, positive effects for us. A personal commitment may be "I am committed to physically training my body. Training clears my mind and builds my physical capacity to deal with what life brings me." When we are personally committed to something, we do the work required to uphold the commitment.

When we commit to our marriage, we metaphorically commit to taking our partner with us wherever we go (Gottman.com Lisa Lund). Would we act differently in certain situations if our partner was with us?

We have the best intentions for our marriage, especially at the time of our wedding vows. Intentions are thoughts and feelings. Commitment is the mindset of doing, taking action, of following through with our intentions. We can say, "I am committed to listening and showing love to my partner." This means we will choose to do the work, day after day, to honor this commitment.

How about committing to our children, with their unique personalities and little isms? Can we turn our good intentions into commitments? Educator and author Robert Ward describes four fundamental aspects of parent commitment:

Leadership – supplies the appropriate guidelines and guidance children require in order to feel a soothing sense of security, structure, and stability.

Love – offers the attention, encouragement, and acceptance that create a strong bond of trust and open communication between adult and child.

Laughter – adds the joy, excitement, and adventure that embolden and assist a child's personal exploration of meaning, purpose, and self-expression.

Learning – develops and reinforces children's knowledge, wisdom, and skills vital for a contributing, self-sufficient life. (Ward October 5, 2016)

CRAWL, WALK, RUN

Ultimate commitment doesn't happen overnight. It is grown, habit by habit, choice by choice. Consider the mantra of crawl, walk, run. When we crawl, we begin with small, daily goals. These are goals that we can easily accomplish, even when we aren't feeling motivated. Little wins provide an incentive to keep going, to move on to our next small goal. As we become proficient at our small goals, we expand to more difficult walking goals. We can keep progressing from there.

As you work on your small goals and start getting into a routine, intentionally assess the process. Are your goals too complex or time-consuming? Are they fairly easy? Could you use more of a challenge? You may need to adjust what you are doing during the process.

COMMITMENT INITIALLY REQUIRES CONSCIOUS EFFORT

At first, we need to make a conscious effort to commit to our practices. Consider scheduling them on your calendar. Once our commitments become habits, we won't need to be so conscious of them. However, to be consistent with our Simplicity tool, we don't want to take on too many commitments at once. Choose one meaningful practice at a time.

Be prepared for your motivation to go through ebbs and flows. We often feel strongly committed to a change or practice at the beginning of our journey. At some point during our progress, we experience a period in which the effort just seems harder. The results don't happen as quickly as we would like. These ebbs and flows are a necessary part of growth. Our resistance is telling us something. When you feel resistance, pay close attention to what triggers it. As you develop your power tool of Awareness, you will be able to identify what is holding you back. When you feel downhearted or frustrated, take a moment to recall why you committed to the practice. This is an opportunity to use some of your other power tools. In what ways can you reframe your thoughts about this practice to ones that are positive? How does this commitment relate to why and how you want to live each day?

TIME FOR CONTEMPLATION

Create some time to specifically think about commitment. Use any mode of reflection that is meaningful to you—prayer, meditation, breathing practice, yoga, walking in nature, etc. After reading the chapter about commitment, what parts resonate with you?

IN YOUR JOURNAL, CONSIDER THE FOLLOWING QUESTIONS:

1. What are your deep-seated reasons for traveling the path of growth and wellness with your spouse and children?

2. What commitments can I begin crawling with?

3. Who do I get to become if I remain committed to my most important goals?

4. What does meaningful and true commitment to my partner look like? How can I put that into action?

5. How can I use the leadership, love, laughter, and learning commitments with my children?

6. Why is this commitment important? What will you and your family gain?

CHAPTER 5

RESILIENCE

"Shit happens, and then you die."
— Tom Taylor (our dad)

Shit does happen. But we don't need to wallow in it. We can grab onto the rope of resilience and pull ourselves back up. Resilience is emotional and mental strength. It's our ability to adapt to and cope with anything that comes our way. This power tool is essential to living fully and courageously. We know that when we make mistakes, miss goals, lose jobs, or lose loved ones, we eventually will be able to get through the situation. It may be painful and uncomfortable, but it will not control our lives. Not only will we survive, but we will become more—more adaptable, more knowledgeable, and more durable.

We can develop, nurture, and strengthen resilience. Resilience won't make a difficult situation go away. We will still feel our emotions. We will still hurt. Resilience will help us see past the experience and realize that life will continue, and we will be able to endure—even if that means enduring a new normal.

HOW DO WE DEVELOP RESILIENCE?

1. By becoming elastic

We need to become elastic—like Elastigirl in the animated film, *The Incredibles*. We must stretch ourselves toward our boundaries, the area just outside of our comfort zone. This area should be uncomfortable but not terrifying. We will likely make mistakes here. But mistakes lead to growth. We can learn from them, take responsibility for them (not play the victim), then slowly release the elastic and recover. Becoming elastic takes daily practice. We stretch ourselves a little further each time, but we don't want to snap like a broken rubber band. When we ease back and recover, we come back stronger (Divine 2020, 190).

2. By becoming flexible

Similar to becoming elastic, we need to become flexible—willing and able to adapt and change according to the challenges. We have to be flexible when we meet a challenge head-on, as well as when we are in the midst of one (Divine 2020, 191). Flexibility involves taking time to assess what is working and what isn't working. We need to be ready to tweak our thoughts and actions at all times.

One way of dealing with a specific challenge does not work for all challenges. Circumstances and conditions are never the same. We need to be physically, mentally, and emotionally flexible.

3. By fully feeling our emotions

We need to feel our emotions. While it is initially easier to avoid painful emotions, avoiding them can destroy us in the future. Uncontrolled sadness, anger, and anxiety are harmful to us and to our relationships. Acknowledging them and working through them is the only way to get to the other side.

4. By becoming durable

We need to become durable, to press on regardless of the circumstances. This may include taking smaller steps forward or reaching out to others for support. Resilient people know that it is okay to ask others for help—asking for help is not a weakness. Having a trusted person to talk to will lighten our load. It will allow us to emerge in better shape than if we tried to do it alone.

Physical durability entails training our body to bounce back and endure. Training stamina (cardiovascular capacity), strength, and flexibility all allow for greater physical resilience. Eating well keeps our gut resilient and our immune system functioning optimally. Sleep and recovery allow for greater long-term endurance and resilience.

5. By becoming positive

A positive, productive attitude is needed to develop resilience. For some reason, many of us think that by anticipating bad situations, we will be ready for them. We won't be surprised or disappointed when they do happen. But this is just inviting negativity into our lives: "Bring it on. I'll be ready." How energy-sucking! Negative energy holds back our potential. It slows our movement forward. A positive attitude invites possibility and creativity. We become solution-oriented. Positivity builds our day-to-day stamina and primes the problem-solving capacity of the mind.

6. By becoming persistent

Persistence is enduring our new-normal over a long period of time. It is emotional control. It requires a daily practice of focus and patience. To stay motivated day-to-day, we need to occasionally divorce ourselves from the end result. We need to focus on the process because we will never quit.

7. By controlling what we can

When we are in the midst of a challenging situation, we want to conserve energy. How do we conserve energy? One way is to focus on what we can control. We then act on what we can control. When we spend time wishing things were different or agonizing over how powerless we feel, we use up our limited supply of energy. It also engages negative energy.

This concept applies to what and how we learn as well. An endless supply of learning opportunities exists in this world. When we are in a challenging situation, we need to prioritize what to learn so we can learn it quickly. Our Simplicity tool applies here. By deciding what is most important and narrowing our focus, we don't lose time and energy by sifting through a pile of impractical information.

HOW DO WE NURTURE AND STRENGTHEN RESILIENCE?

To nurture our resilience, we need to keep our battery fully charged. This means we need to take care of ourselves; we need to keep ourselves healthy. Self-care includes having good quality sleep, eating healthy food, drinking plenty of water, moving our bodies, spending time outside, and practicing our breathing. If a challenge should appear, we will be fully functioning and ready to address it head-on.

Resilience gets strengthened every time we use it. It is like a mental and emotional muscle. Similar to building muscles, developing resilience is uncomfortable. If we notice a particular trigger or feeling of resistance, let's pay close attention to it. The trigger is highlighting something. What is holding us back? As we continue to practice resistance, we'll find that we can progressively push ourselves a little further. So, the next time we fall down, we will get back up even stronger than before.

Various traditions and religions discuss how to address challenges—by letting go, by practicing non-attachment, and by putting them in God's hands. They highlight that our life experiences are neither good nor bad. They just are. We attach meaning to situations and label them as good or bad. Think of the thumbs-up sign we give our kids to acknowledge and encourage them. We've attached a positive meaning to the gesture. If we gave a thumbs-up sign to someone in the Middle East, it would be like giving them the middle finger, essentially saying, "Up yours!" A negative meaning has been attached to the same gesture. Without the attached meaning, our thumb is simply a body part.

During a future challenging situation, let's take a moment to practice the tool of Awareness. What meaning have we attached to the situation? Do we want to continue down the path of suffering, or do we want to choose a path toward peace? By practicing non-attachment, we realize that the challenges don't define us or become us. We don't need to dwell on them. They simply become a line of text in our narrative instead of a significant, destructive plot twist in an otherwise beautiful story.

Resilience can turn the biggest mess into the most powerful message. Struggle is okay. It enriches our lives and helps us continue to grow. Both marriage and parenting provide the ultimate training grounds to learn resilience. We mess up over and over again, but we get up the next day and try to do it better.

TIME FOR CONTEMPLATION

Create some time to specifically think about resilience. Use any mode of reflection that is meaningful to you—prayer, meditation, breathing practice, yoga, walking in nature, etc. After reading the chapter about resilience, what parts resonate with you?

IN YOUR JOURNAL, CONSIDER THE FOLLOWING QUESTIONS:

1. Consider the obstacles that you've overcome in the past. Name them.

2. What process did you use to overcome them? How can the skills you've developed to overcome be optimized?

3. Can you think of family obstacles or current situations that still control your thoughts?

4. What language can you use to view challenges through a positive, growth-oriented lens?

CHAPTER 6

AWARENESS

"Awareness is the greatest agent for change."
- Eckhart Tolle

Awareness is a powerful tool that creates space and understanding. Awareness gives us a chance to respond instead of react. We respond more thoughtfully and purposefully, often seeking clarification. Awareness is the act of noticing— without forming judgments or assumptions.

This. Is. Not. Easy.

Our brains crave meaning, wanting to associate actions with meanings. In fact, this is how memories are made. But awareness is not about putting down memories. Awareness involves noticing and examining a thought, feeling, or action before forming a memory. It will take practice. Luckily, we have so many opportunities to practice this power tool simply within our family.

Awareness is self-examination on steroids. It involves understanding ourselves on a deeper level. With self-awareness, we explore our subconscious mind and notice our thoughts and feelings. This is metacognition in action again—the process of identifying and evaluating our thoughts. About ninety percent of our thoughts during the day come from our subconscious mind. But what are they? Do we want to operate in this way, live according to an unexamined mind? Retired Navy SEAL Commander Mark Divine describes this as "connecting with our witness self" (Divine 2015, 26). We witness our thoughts. What is going on inside there? What are we saying to ourselves? We begin to see thoughts not as something that belong to us, rather as something passing, impermanent.

Metacognition is just one branch of self-awareness. Another branch that sprouts from self-awareness is somatic awareness. (Somatic is a fancy Latin word meaning "related to the body.") This involves noticing sensations in our body. Do we feel hungry or full? Do we feel tightness anywhere? How about pain or discomfort? Somatic awareness also consists of our senses—taste, smell, sight, sound, touch. What do we notice? We will explore somatic awareness in more detail in Section ll.

Emotional awareness is the third branch of self-awareness. It involves paying attention to what we are feeling. We notice our emotions without judgment. Negative feelings such as anger or jealousy are hard to notice without judging at first. But we can take small steps. Let's begin by simply focusing on our emotions—without worrying about whether or not we are judging them. Can we simply name the emotions as they are felt? When we are proficient at this, we can add in the practice of non-judgment. For example, we notice that we feel jealous when our neighbors upgrade their minivan to the latest Porsche SUV. We feel our emotions but aren't yet able to separate them from judgment. "What a doofus! Why the hell would they buy that kind of vehicle when they have young kids? How will my 1985 wood-paneled station wagon look parked next to that thing?" Baby steps. In this case, we are still clearly in the early phase of noticing our emotions.

The fourth branch of self-awareness is pattern or habit awareness. This involves paying attention to our habits in our daily lives. It is estimated that up to ninety percent of our daily activities are based on habits. Do we know what our habits are? We will initially work at noticing and identifying our habits. Again, we will do so without judgment or blame. Once we become aware of our habits or patterns, we can choose whether we want to maintain them, let them go, or replace them with a healthier option. We will further explore habit awareness in the upcoming chapters.

As we grow in our self-awareness, we can extend our practice of awareness to interactions with our family. In order to deepen our relationships with our family members, what can we pay attention to? What can we focus on? Are they telling us something without being able to find the words? Interpersonal awareness is noticing a person's partly expressed language, such as body language, tone of voice, and other subtle mannerisms. We don't want to judge or make assumptions when we use interpersonal awareness. Let's just notice, then ask for clarification, such as when talking with our child, "I noticed that you rolled your eyes when I asked you to make your bed. What did you mean by that?" Asking for clarification also teaches our children that it is okay to pause, to think, then connect their thoughts to their actions.

As we continue to discuss awareness, it is important to note that we humans are great storytellers. These are beyond the stories we tell around the campfire. These are narratives that go on inside of our heads. We subconsciously tie our own unique narrative to facts and occurrences. Each of us creates narratives based on past experiences and feelings—they become our perspective. We do it so quickly that we think everyone should believe our narrative-laced truth. For example, imagine you and your partner observe the same incident: Your child drops to the floor in the middle of the grocery store, assumes a face-down, snow-angel position, and starts screaming. Those are the facts. A story occurs when we add our narrative to the facts. You think I knew Frodo had anger issues. He has been acting out more frequently lately. He probably inherited his issues from his grandfather—ugh, so I have him to thank. I'll need to call a therapist as soon as we get home. Your partner, who witnessed the same event, thinks Our little Frodo is hungry and exhausted. We need to get him home, feed him a healthy meal, and get him to bed early tonight. He'll be his happy-go-lucky self in the morning. You and your partner both claim to have been fully aware of the situation. Is one perspective better than the other perspective? Is it surprising that most conflicts arise from the difference in our stories rather than the facts hidden somewhere within the stories? As we continue to practice awareness, we will become better equipped at noticing our narratives.

Breathing, mindfulness, meditation, and somatic practices are all conduits to deep awareness. They give our brain a chance to rest and be quiet. This allows us to tune in to our thought patterns and narratives. We will learn more about the specific types of awareness and how they relate to our Self in Sections ll through lV.

TIME FOR CONTEMPLATION

Create time to specifically think about awareness. Use any mode of reflection that is meaningful to you—prayer, meditation, breathing practice, yoga, walking in nature, etc. After reading the chapter about awareness, what parts resonate with you?

IN YOUR JOURNAL, CONSIDER THE FOLLOWING QUESTIONS:

1. What thought patterns do I currently notice that I'd like to change?

2. What patterns do I have that I'd love to grow?

3. What are my daily habits? Are there any that I'd like to change? Why?

4. What internal language do I use when thinking about my partner? Does it support us having a loving relationship?

5. Am I aware of attempts my partner makes to express love? What are they? How do I respond?

6. Think of a recent disconnect you had with your partner. Did you each have a different narrative about the situation?

7. For each child, what do you notice when they try to convey a message without using words?

For each child, consider assumptions you make about their behavior. Could your assumptions be inaccurate? If your children are school-age or older, ask them what they hope to accomplish with that behavior.

CHAPTER 7

PURPOSE

There is a "you-shaped" hole in the universe.
— Caroline McHugh

Our passion. Our mission. Our practice. Personally meaningful. Positively affects others. And multi-layered. Together, these describe Purpose. All too often, we think we need to find our purpose like it is something lurking around the corner just out of our reach. Or we think we must endure a life-altering experience—something that screams, "Wake up! Behold, your purpose!" If you've experienced such an experience, how wonderful. And how rare. The rest of us connect with our purpose in a simpler manner, realized in everyday moments.

Think about the phrases "on purpose" and "by accident." They are opposites on the spectrum. So, how do we want to live each day—on purpose or by accident? Do we want to be in the driver's seat, or do we want to face backward in the rear seat of the old station wagon? If by accident, we find ourselves in the back of the two-toned cruiser, sucking in its exhaust, we can only see where we've been. Life feels like it is happening to us or around us. We spend our time reacting to stimuli, hitting our heads on the ceiling with every unexpected bump in the road. Why are we choosing this? How would we rather travel? If we want to live on purpose, we need to turn around, crawl over the two rows of seats, and grab onto the steering wheel.

Purpose provides meaning and guidance in our day-to-day lives. It is why and how we choose to live. We experience deeper growth and fulfillment when we match our why and how to what we do in our lives. Our "what" includes our choice of profession, our lifestyle. If we don't tie the three together, something feels "off." If we continue down that path without consciously taking action, it can lead to anxiety and depression. For example, Sven is a medical doctor. He has a reputable title and earns a decent salary. His purpose is to provide care for his patients as if they were members of his own family. However, his clinic time with each patient is strictly limited to ten minutes regardless of the patients' symptoms. At work, he doesn't feel able to fully live his purpose. Yet, he endures his clinic practice. From the outside, Sven looks like he has it all. In reality, Sven is restless, angry, and often irritable. His unfulfillment at work affects the way he lives his purpose at home. It is hard to practice "caring for his family" when he is so impatient and on edge. After talking with a therapist for several months, Sven decided to work part-time at the clinic. He also began to volunteer for an organization that provides medical care to underserved people. No time restrictions for patient care. No salary provided. But a new, deeply enriched sense of self, work, and family. His why and how he wanted to live matched what he did in his day-to-day life.

PURPOSE AS OUR LIFE'S THEME

Purpose is a predominant life-serving ambition, such as, "I want to live a healthy, balanced life—physically, mentally, and spiritually." Our lives are like multi-volume novels, similar to the Harry Potter® series of books. Each book is divided into chapters—chapters that involve challenges, mysteries, plot twists, and discoveries. Like our lives, a novel usually includes someone or something worth protecting. Though each novel in a multi-volume series has its own storyline, one strong principal theme is often woven throughout the volumes. The theme is a recurring idea, an essential part of the books that guides the reader forward. In the Harry Potter® series, a foundational theme is the fear of death and the unknown— yet when the characters faced their fear of it, they could more fully experience life. Purpose is our personal life theme. It guides us in our day-to-day lives. Throughout our lives, our storylines will change. Circumstances and experiences will influence our lives. Some may even feel like major turning points. But does our foundational purpose change? No, it does not. Its shape may change, or a limb may be added, but our foundation remains firm.

WHY IS PURPOSE IMPORTANT?

Purpose provides value and significance now. As we know, our purpose is not a one-stop destination. With purpose, we live each day consciously and with intention. We make deliberate, thoughtful choices that shape our lives. What shape will eventually be formed; we are not sure. And does it matter? Our journey is where we make our choices, act out our purpose, and write our story. Choices are like dots in a complicated, adult dot-to-dot puzzle. We journey along the dots until, ultimately, a beautiful picture is revealed. During our travels, we wondered where the dots were leading or if we missed a few of them. Connecting the dots serves a greater purpose— to create a work of art. We connect the dots in our daily lives by deciding what to do, how to move forward. We often don't see the bigger picture, especially during the difficult parts of our journey. It's only when we look back, through our life's straight and circuitous routes, that we comprehend how the dots united to create our Self—a unique work of art.

By living with purpose, we have a chance to live a happier, healthier, and longer life. Since our energy is directed toward something positive, our brain releases healthy chemicals that fuel and strengthen our bodies. Researchers found that "a higher sense of purpose correlates to reduced risks of disability, stroke, heart disease, sleep issues, and other health problems" (Chen et al. 2019, 664). So, we can live longer, healthier lives with a deeper sense of meaning. What are we waiting for?

HOW DO WE CULTIVATE OUR PURPOSE?

Cultivating our purpose can sound intimidating. Rest assured, most of us are already living at least some aspects of our purpose without knowing it. We simply don't know how to put it into words, how to fill in the blank, "My purpose is ____." We continue to cultivate this life practice through deliberate action and reflection. During reflection, think about the following questions:

- What are your strengths? What do other people appreciate about you? We are not talking about your physique or your clothing style. These are superficial and not sustaining. Do people appreciate the way you listen, pay attention to them, or make them laugh? Think about why you do you those things.

- Is there something meaningful you would like to do to improve the lives of others? Have you experienced pain or suffering that you don't want others to experience?

- Have you read any books that spurred a passion in you? Reading helps us learn about ourselves, even if it is a fiction novel. You may find information or characters that awaken your purpose. Even characters in a fiction novel can provide insight into values and purpose.

CAN OUR CHILDREN CULTIVATE PURPOSE?

Children spend much of their time exploring their environment. They discover their likes and dislikes without having a deep motive other than to play. William Damon, author of The Path to Purpose describes purpose as a "chemical reaction that occurs when our skills meet the needs of the world. Eventually, young people identify something in their environment that could be improved. With some added maturity, they are able to recognize something within themselves that could help solve that problem" (Damon 2009, 162). When young people get to know their skills and interests, they start to pursue their purpose. Not so different from adults.

Cultivating our purpose doesn't have an endpoint by which we need to have everything figured out. Remember that finding and living our purpose are steps on our journey—not a destination. We just have to be willing to explore what skills we have and what deeply matters to us.

TIME FOR CONTEMPLATION

Create time to specifically think about purpose. What values are important to you? Use any mode of reflection that is meaningful to you—prayer, meditation, breathing practice, yoga, walking in nature, etc. After reading the chapter about purpose, what parts resonate with you?

IN YOUR JOURNAL, CONSIDER THE FOLLOWING QUESTIONS, THEN ASK YOURSELF, "WHY?"

1. What do I like to do in my free time?

2. When do I feel the most satisfied?

3. How can I use my talents to be of service?

4. When I was a child, what did I love to do?

5. Are there specific experiences I feel have shaped me as a person?

6. What do I want my life to be defined as?

7. What will be written in my obituary?

8. What is your purpose as a couple? Does your purpose affect others, or does it mainly apply to you two?

9. Name your children's strengths.

10. Ask your children what they feel their strengths are. Ask them what things they like to do for others.

11. Ask your children, "If you had a day with absolutely no plans, what would you do?"

Does your family have a purpose? Does the purpose apply just to your family, or does it affect others?

BREATH PRACTICE

We have mentioned breath practice as a tool for cultivating the character power tools. It will continue to be an important practice moving forward. If breath practice is new to you, here is a simple way to start.

4 Simple Steps

1. Take a Seat
2. Breathe
3. Concentrate
4. Take Notice

STEP 1:

Take a Seat

- Begin by sitting upright
- Sit on the floor with legs crossed, on the edge of a chair or meditation bench.
- Sit comfortably enough that your body position is not a distraction.

Aim to sit tall

- When the spine is long, the core is active and energy flows through the spinal column.
- Allow palms to rest gently on thighs or knees.

- Welcome to your breath practice position.

Tips:

Sit on a bolster or blanket if hips are tight or flexibility is limited.

Visualize a thread being pulled through the crown of the head to lengthen the spine. A small tuck of the tailbone and chin can also help.

STEP 2:

Breathe

- Begin inhaling and exhaling through the nose.
- Regardless of the pattern of breath, the goal will always be to fill the lungs fully.
- Feel the diagram expand. Allow core muscles to soften on inhale and engage to assist exhale.
- Aim to feel air move from the nostrils

Patterns

- Centering: Match length of deep inhale and exhale (consider 5 seconds for each to start).
- Calming: brief inhale with twice as long exhale. Example: 5 second inhale, 10 second exhale.
- Energizing: quick inhale and exhale (still full breath, though)

- There are many more but these are awesome patterns to start with!

STEP 3:

Concentrate

Focus on breath

- Begin to breathe deeply. How does the breath feel entering and leaving the lungs? Can you feel the diaphragm expand and contract? How soft can the edges of the breath be (the brief moment between inhale and exhale)? Watch the breath and the sensations that go along with it.

- The pattern of breathing, such as the inhale and exhale to a count, can also be a point of concentration.

Use Mantra

- Using words as a point of focus is another great way to build concentration power. Prayer is a mantra. A positive statement like "I am healthier and better every day" is mantra. Repeating one word like "Om" is mantra. Pick something that resonates with you.

Pick an Object

- Light a candle and focus on the flame. Look at a favorite picture. Use a religious item that resonates with you like a cross or holy book. Stabilizing attention on the object is concentration.

Tips:

- The idea is to use your attention to stay focused on the object of concentration. The awesome thing is that your attention will drift from this object and when you notice the attention shift, you can recognize it! This is awareness.

- You might begin to notice a certain type of thought (judgement, fear, etc). Notice it and return to your object of concentration. As we begin to be able to watch our thoughts instead of be our thoughts, major shifts can happen.

STEP 4:

Take Notice

As we refine our ability to concentrate, we begin to build our ability to witness what is happening in our own mind and body.

We can begin to recognize patterns of thought. We can recognize the story of who we were raised to be and how that compares to who we really are.

Instead of being our stream of thoughts (which we have more than 50,000 thoughts per day), we can see thoughts as a flow of information—some true, some not—that change like the wind.

We can examine thoughts without being attached to the thought or emotion behind it. Being able to witness thought is serious business. Like life changing business.

The hope is not to be thoughtless but curious about our thoughts. In control of thoughts. Unattached to thoughts.

You also might begin to experience space between thoughts. For example, you may be repeating a mantra and then notice for a brief moment you were not repeating the mantra or thinking about anything else. Enjoy those brief moments of bliss and what might become available to you in those moments.

Space between thought contains so much information that we suck up like a vacuum. It doesn't require processing or interpretation. It is universal intelligence, God, whatever you want to call it. It is the awesome sauce of regular, consistent practice.

Wherever you are, meet yourself there. If you are just getting started, great! If you have practiced for years but hit a roadblock, no problem.

Breath practice isn't a pass or fail activity. We aren't winning medals. We are steadily connecting to ourselves in our highest form.

SECTION II
THE PHYSICAL SELF

Here we go! We have the tools—now let's begin building our foundation. Our physical body supports all that we are. Cultures and religions throughout the ages have described the physical self as our foundation, our vessel, our armor. We build and refine the rest of ourselves from there.

Psychologist Abraham Maslow described human needs that must be met in order to evolve. To evolve means to grow and develop, to become the best possible version of ourselves. Maslow is the creator of the well-known hierarchy of needs. The base of the pyramid is our physical needs: food, shelter, air, water, clothing, sleep. Our foundation. His theory is that in order to deepen our awareness and move on to the next levels of ourselves, we need to first meet most of our physical needs (Maslow 1970).

As we will see, practices that apply to our physical Self carry over and affect our mental and spiritual Selves as well. Yet, each aspect of our Selves affects the other two. Since our physical Self is our base, it needs to be strong. This is done through movement. To maintain its strength, our physical Self needs to be made of high-quality materials. This is done through healthy nutrition. A healthy base will allow our other aspects of Self to function optimally. For example, if we lie around every day eating snack cakes and Doritos® (our physical Self), the lack of movement and questionable nutrition affects how we process information (our mental Self). It also affects our ability to breathe deeply and concentrate on our inner thoughts (our spiritual Self). We are just too bloated, and our blood sugar level is through the roof.

Realizing the need for a strong physical foundation, let's try to shift our focus from how our body looks to what our body can do. What is it capable of? How well does it function? Can we physically do all that we want to do?

In the Physical Self section, we will describe the importance of Movement and Nutrition, and how to put them into practice—ideas for you personally, for your marriage, and for the whole family. We will also share how each of the Power Tools we covered in the last section can be used to strengthen Movement and Nutrition. This section is not a fitness plan or a special diet. We will give you examples of movement and nutrition plans to guide you, but you need to ultimately decide how to make them personal and meaningful for you. Finally, we will provide some action steps to try regardless of where you currently are on your journey.

This is the one body we have to live in—if we care for it, stand by; the trajectory for the rest of our Self is limitless!

CHAPTER 8

MOVEMENT

Movement is action. It is a powerful, inexpensive medicine. Moving our body on a regular basis positively affects our whole body. It improves our sleep, increases our energy, increases our strength and flexibility, increases our mental functioning, and reduces pain and stress. Movement benefits every aspect of our Self!

Movement is more than exercise; more than a structured, repetitive approach to getting in better physical shape. The focus of movement is to become physically capable and more durable—so we can fully participate in our lives. It involves a greater awareness of how physical activity affects our body. Movement consists of both structured and unstructured activities, including exercise, play, and day-to-day physical tasks. And the simplest movement of all is breathing. It is also one of the most powerful. It helps us become mindful of the process. We will bring our body and mind together to strengthen our commitment to our new lifestyle. We will become mindful bodies in motion.

MOVEMENT HELPS US PHYSICALLY FUNCTION BETTER

Movement develops our muscle groups and cardiovascular capacity—our heart, lungs, and blood vessels. We move to train ourselves for day-to-day activities, for real-life situations. Our lives are made up of complex movements. We don't work in the yard using only our triceps. We don't pick up our children with just our hands. Movement is a practice in coordination, strength, and endurance. Daily movement prepares our body for running, bending, and stooping; and to actively play with our children and protect them from harm. What if our daughter Hortense stumbles on a family hike, falls down a steep hill, and injures her ankle? Are we able to side-step down the hill, pick up fifty-pound Hortense, and carry her up the hill and back to the car? Or do we slide down the hill on our backside and wait for help to hopefully arrive? If we want to be strong and capable, and give our family our best Self, let's make daily movement a priority. It is training for our health, for our family's wellbeing, and for life itself.

Movement improves our quality of life, but does it affect the quantity of time we have yet to live? It just may. A widely reported study involved a test devised by Brazilian physicians and researchers in exercise and sports medicine. Study volunteers were asked to sit down on the floor and then get up, using the least amount of support from their hands, knees, elbows, and other body parts. The volunteers received a perfect ten if they were able to sit and stand without any support. Points were deducted for each body part that they leaned on when trying to sit or stand. After studying 2,002 adults over an average of six years, one of the physician researchers, Dr. Araujo stated, "It is well-known that aerobic fitness is strongly related to survival, but our study also shows that maintaining high levels of body flexibility, muscle strength, [muscle] power-to-body weight ratio and coordination are not only good for performing daily activities, but have a favorable influence on life expectancy" (Brito, L. B.B. et al. 2012). He said the test quickly rated how well a person physically functioned from day to day. While this is only one study, a number of other studies have shown the relationship between movement and a higher quality of life. The bottom line is that in order to function well in life, we need to move regularly—movement that includes aerobic exercise, muscle strengthening, flexibility, and balance. This is training for life.

What if our bodies could physically change depending on the environment we created for them? It sounds like something out of a science-fiction movie. But it's not. Our bodies do physically change according to certain environments. Think about how common it used to be to intentionally or unintentionally interact with people who smoked. We could be sitting in a restaurant enjoying our dinner while the patrons behind us enjoyed their Camels® and their Marlboros®. We, in turn, inhaled their smoke. It was not unusual to see a smokey haze hovering near the ceiling in many restaurants and bars. We now know that an environment filled with passive smoke can change our body—our lungs in particular. As a result, most of us choose not to subject our bodies to that environment.

What type of environment are we exposing our bodies to today?

Sitting.

Our bodies were not designed to sit for long periods of time. We were designed to stand and move. Have you heard the tagline, "Sitting is the new smoking?" A number of studies show that sitting for more than eight hours a day without any physical activity carries a similar risk of dying as smoking and obesity. (Lakerfield et al. 2017, 77) The inactivity itself raises our risk of obesity, diabetes, heart disease, and deep vein thrombosis (blood clots), not to mention the adverse mental effects it has on us. At least we are not spewing carcinogens into the air, affecting the lungs of those around us. However, if we sit most of the day, day after day, we actually do affect the lives of others. We affect how much we can physically do with those that matter to us, such as our partner and children.

When we sit most of the day, our body changes. Specific muscles tighten and get shorter. Tight hip flexor muscles and hamstrings can cause low back pain. These muscle changes also affect our gait and our balance. Our joints get stiff. Our gluteal (butt) muscles become weak. Our spinal column compresses. And we feel pain. However, many of us can't get away from sitting with the type of work that we do. What options do we have?

We can build short movement breaks into our schedule. Taking quick breaks to move frequently throughout the day can counteract the many effects of sitting. These breaks benefit our body much more than being inactive during the workweek, then doing a weekend grind at the gym.

What are some examples of movement activities for those of us that sit most of the day?

- Set an alarm to move every thirty minutes. Do some air squats, walk around, walk up and down the stairs, or even do some push-ups.
- Stand or walk around when you talk on the phone.
- Stand when you read your e-mails.
- Try having a meeting with someone while walking.
- Rather than sitting down to read, listen to an audiobook while taking a walk or working outside.

You can also consider using a standing desk or improvise by elevating your laptop on a box (on your desk) or work at a standing-height counter.

We each have our own personal reasons for moving and staying strong. Yet, we all want to move with the most efficient body possible. Daily practice and consistency are more important than fixating on the final result, such as a better physique or weight loss. If we focus on our practice and its daily benefits, the results will come. We will feel so much better—we'll wonder how we lived without it!

JAKE'S DISCOVERY OF THE CRAWL, WALK, RUN MANTRA

After a major life transition going from a professional athlete to an office job, Jake had to learn how to navigate his days without built-in workouts. He had been doing regular cardiovascular training and muscle strengthening movements as part of hockey practice since he was four years old. What happened when he transitioned to a sitting profession? He recalls a family gathering during this time in which he was sitting on the couch with his dad. He felt sad and irritable. And guilty. Here he was surrounded by his most loving support system—his immediate family and family of origin—but couldn't give any part of himself to them. This dark place was not where he wanted to stay. A thought popped into his head as he sat observing his family's intergenerational activities. What is one thing I can control right now? I can move my body. I don't feel like moving, but I will use some of my dormant resiliency skills and go for a ten-minute run. That was his turning point. A simple, doable decision. He gradually increased his running miles. After just a week, he felt a little stronger, more confident, and more courageous to take on something new. He signed up at a local Cross-Fit gym. And the rest is history. He continues his Cross-Fit workouts to this day and is now a Cross-Fit Level 1 trainer. Jake says, "I was the only limiting factor in my health and fitness." He attributes the majority of his success to his mantra of crawl, walk, run.

We can compare our movement training to our development from an infant to a child. We first learned to control our movements. We then learned to crawl, then walk, and finally, we learned to run. We will use a similar method to build our strength. We will perfect each movement one by one until it creates a strong foundation for the next one. When we have a setback, we are reassured that we have a strong base. We don't have to start all over again. Let's remember to give ourselves love and patience to progress at our own speed, as long as we move daily.

MOVEMENT AND THE BLUE ZONES

Dan Buettner studied specific areas of the world in which the longest-living people resided. He called these the Blue Zones of happiness and longevity. Not only did these people live such long lives, but they also had a high quality of life— still living at home, playing games, gathering socially, and having sex. On the whole, they were healthy and exhibited a very low rate of dementia. What made them live such long and fulfilling lives? Buettner and his research team found nine common denominators in all of the Blue Zones. One of the nine lifestyle habits was moving naturally. Buettner said, "The world's longest-living people don't pump iron, run marathons, or join gyms. Instead, they live in environments that constantly nudge them into moving without thinking about it. They grow gardens and don't have mechanical conveniences for house and yard work" (Buettner 2012, 34). Residents in the blue zones moved all day, at an average of every twenty minutes. These amazing people were in their eighties and nineties, and many were centenarians! So, with our robotic vacuums and house in the suburbs, how can we find innovative ways to move?

Cole's awareness of her need for movement changed when her kids were young. Though she had frequented gyms as a young adult, exercise was more about fitting into her jeans and less about how it made her feel. With young children, she often felt drained, was easily exhausted, and felt somewhat aimless. She attributed these feelings to trying to survive in a busy child-rearing period. One day during this time, as she was giving the kids a bath, she decided to start some type of movement. She proceeded to do ten push-ups against the bathtub. Another simple, doable decision. By the time the kids were done playing in the tub, she had done three sets of ten push-ups. She opted to do some simple movements like this every day. Within a short timespan, she noticed that the fog was lifting from her brain.

We can all find ways to increase our movements throughout the day. We can get up and walk to talk to a family member in another area of the house—rather than yell or text them. We can have a race with our kids. We can park farther away from our destination and walk the rest of the way. We can take the stairs. Or we can put the kids in the bathtub and do some push-ups.

MOVEMENT AND BRAIN HEALTH

If it isn't enough that movement provides increased strength, function, and a longer life, how about improving our mood, focus, and memory? An amazing relationship exists between movement and the health of our brain.

Movement protects our brain.

Movement creates positive changes in our brain.

Movement even grows our brain!

When we move and get our heart pumping, more oxygen-rich blood flows to our brain. It stimulates the release of chemicals called growth factors. These powerhouse chemicals send out signals to grow new blood vessels in the brain. They help develop new brain cells. Neural connections are also increased—to link and support the new brain cells, as well as to protect our current ones. A lot happens in our brain with regular movement, so let's look at one area that is vastly affected by such activity.

The hippocampus is an area deep within the brain. Learning and the formation of long-term memories occur here. The hippocampus is the first area of the brain to become damaged due to Alzheimer's Disease. With regular aerobic activity, new brain cells and connections form in this area—the volume of the hippocampus actually increases. The hippocampus grows! This increases our capacity for learning and long-term memories. It also adds protection from dementia and Alzheimer's disease (Basso, Suzuki 2017). Many studies have shown that with regular physical activity, other brain regions that contribute to thinking and memory also increase in volume. Neuroscientist Dr. Scott McGinnis says that within six to twelve months of regular physical activity, we can increase the volume of our entire brain (McGinnis 2021).

Aerobic movement can indirectly affect our brain by reducing inflammation in our body. You may have heard of "inflammatory diseases" or "chronic inflammation." Stress, smoking, obesity, and regular alcohol use contribute to chronic inflammation. Chronic inflammation essentially causes a constant message of high alert in our body. This can lead to damage to our body's organs—including the brain. Our growth factors can't signal as effectively. They are less capable of growing new brain cells and protecting the ones that we have. Diabetes, high blood pressure, and heart disease are examples of inflammatory diseases. Though we don't think of these as brain diseases, they play a part in brain and nerve damage. This is where movement comes to the rescue again—movement reduces inflammation in the body and the brain.

Another indirect effect that movement has on our brain is improving our mood. Aerobic movement reduces stress and anxiety. It helps us sleep better. Stress, anxiety, and lack of sleep all lead to a decline in brain function. The good news is that our brain makes and stores chemicals that relieve anxiety and depression and promote sleep. They just need some help to be released into our body. Physical activity acts as a key to unlock and release our big three mood regulators—dopamine, serotonin, and norepinephrine. These chemical messengers in the brain are called neurotransmitters. They improve our memory, our reaction times, and our ability to concentrate.

And they begin to work immediately after physical activity. Their effects can last for two to three hours after the activity!

Consider the emotions of our children, especially after they've endured a long day at school. When their emotions run high, we can show them how to use movement to help them regulate their energy. Decide to leave the homework on the table and go play a game of tag.

So, physical activity can literally change our brain. As neuroscientist Wendy Suzuki said,

> What if I could give you something that would have immediate, positive benefits for your brain, including your mood and your focus? And what if I told you that same thing could actually last a long time and protect your brain from different conditions like depression, Alzheimer's disease and dementia? Yes. I am talking about the powerful effects of physical activity. Simply moving your body has immediate, long-lasting, protective benefits for your brain that can last for the rest of your life. (Suzuki 0:15)

HOW OFTEN SHOULD WE MOVE?

The National Institutes of Health recommend that adults get at least 150 minutes of physical activity in a week. But we can move much more often than that. We know that every type of movement counts toward our health. Our children and teens should get at least an hour of physical activity per day—another opportunity for us to move and connect with our kids. Ready for a game of flashlight tag or Marco Polo in the pool?

COLE'S EMOTIONAL ENCOUNTER WITH CRAWL, WALK, RUN

Cole grew up playing sports. She didn't realize how directly her physical activity added to her sense of well-being. She just knew that she enjoyed freely moving her body and was able to effortlessly do a wide range of activities. At age nineteen, Cole had to suddenly stop all physical activities—she was struck by a drunk driver in a head-on collision. She endured a long recovery. Before the accident, her movement of choice was running. After the accident, running was only a pipe dream. Using the Crawl, Walk, Run mantra, she began to crawl. Her first movement of choice became walking in a pool.

Not only did she feel the physical effects of her injuries, but she also felt the mental and emotional effects. She wasn't getting regular boosts of neurotransmitters—her internal mood regulators. Since she had a history of being physically active, she discovered the link between lack of movement and her diminished mood and concentration. She had learned what it felt like to be in shape before she knew the feeling of being out of shape. This was a wake-up call to her. She didn't like the physical or emotional aspects of being out of shape. She was determined to find doable movements while allowing her body to recover. Thankfully, we are all capable of moving in one way or another, even if the activity won't be featured on the cover of Sports Illustrated.

MOVEMENT AND THE VAGUS NERVE

Aerobic movement and deep abdominal breathing reduce anxiety and chronic inflammation. They help us feel calm and think more clearly. One way they accomplish this is by stimulating the vagus nerve (Gerritsen, Band 2018). When stress hormones send us into fight-or-flight—our sympathetic nervous system, our saber-toothed tiger reaction, the vagus nerve is responsible for getting us into our rest-and-recover response—our parasympathetic nervous system. This system returns our body back to a steady state after being in fight-or-flight mode. It reduces our heart rate, slows our breathing, and allows us to digest our food properly. It calms our body.

So, what does this have to do with the brain? The vagus nerve starts in the brain. It is the longest nerve in our body, traveling from our brain all the way to our gut. This multi-function nerve contains branches like a tree that connect it to the heart, lungs, and other major organs. It functions as a communication superhighway.

Our body is only designed to be in fight-or-flight mode for a short period of time. In its high alert state, our body releases stress hormones that supply it with immediate energy—adrenaline and cortisol. Adrenaline increases our heart rate and blood pressure. Cortisol increases our blood sugar and slows the function of our digestive system and other body systems that aren't needed to fight or flee. A toned vagus nerve quickly brings our body systems back to a steady state after the threat is gone. Our heart rate and blood pressure return to normal, our blood sugar decreases, and we have full use of our brain again.

Our body can overreact to stressors that are not life-threatening but are always present. In this case, our natural alarm system stays turned on. This is the red zone, the danger zone. Stress hormones continue to surge, contributing all of their effects to our body. We can't remain healthy in this state for an extended time. Long-term exposure to stress hormones is also known as chronic stress. It can cause a number of health conditions, such as depression, anxiety, brain fog, digestive problems, weight gain, and headaches. It also leads to inflammatory diseases such as heart disease, diabetes, and some types of cancers.

Each of us perceives and reacts to life's stressors in different ways. Regardless, we overestimate the stressor and underestimate our ability to cope with it. Due to the dangerous health risks of chronic stress, we want to identify and manage our stressors. We need to course-correct.

STRENGTHENING OUR VAGUS NERVE TONE

We can strengthen our vagus nerve tone through physical activity and deep breathing.

1. Deep breathing exercises. This is one of the most effective ways to stimulate our vagus nerve. And we can do it any time at any location. Slowly inhale to a

count of five, hold for a count of five, slowly exhale for a count of five, hold for a count of five. Then repeat.

2. Yoga. Yoga asanas, the movements and postures of yoga, increase tone of the vagus nerve. Coordinating these movements with deep breathing is a powerhouse combination. In addition to deep breathing, another way to quickly stimulate the vagus nerve is in a forward fold. Simply reaching for your toes from a standing position can trigger the vagus nerve to activate the parasympathetic nervous system.

3. Singing and humming. These activities cause vibrations that stimulate the vagus nerve. The vibrations reduce and help us move from our fight-or-flight mode to rest and digest mode.

4. Laughing. This causes vibrations that stimulate the vagus nerve. The unexpected side effects of laughing— coughing, urinating, passing gas—also contribute to strengthening the nerve.

5. Cold exposure. Try splashing your face with cold water. You may eventually progress to taking a cold shower. Try a polar bear plunge with your partner. Go roll in the snow, then jump in a hot tub with your kids.

6. In essence, every time we take a deep abdominal breath, with or without movement, we stimulate our vagus nerve. This benefits our whole Self, connecting our physical, mental, and spiritual Self.

MOVEMENT AND RECOVERY WITH LOVING KINDNESS

As part of developing awareness of our physical body, we need to pay attention to signs of fatigue. Are you feeling unusually tired? Do you feel uncoordinated? Do movements that usually feel easy to you feel challenging? It is important to balance days in which we do long or intense physical activity with days of gentle, recovery movements. Recovery allows our muscles to heal. Recovery movements promote blood flow to our muscles, increase flexibility, and relieve tight areas. Recovery movements include tai chi, gentle yoga, stretching, and foam-rolling, easy swimming, walking, or biking. If we grind or engage in intense physical activity day after day without listening to our body, we won't perform as well. In fact, we expose ourselves to toxic stress and high cortisol levels, similar to being in a continual state of fight-or-flight. As we know, this can hurt our body, and our brain can't function as well if it persists in this state.

Recovery also includes getting adequate sleep, drinking plenty of water, and fueling our body with healthy food. Have you heard about sleep recharging your battery? Recharging our brain is essentially what sleep does. It replenishes our energy, helps improve our performance, releases hormones that help our muscles and brain recover, and positively influences our body's response to stress and nutrition. As neuroscientist Dr. Matthew Walker stated, "Sleep is probably the greatest legal performance-enhancing drug that few are abusing enough" (Walker 2018).

HOW ARE PHYSICAL HEALTH AND MOVEMENT REFLECTED IN TRADITIONS?

The thousand-plus-year tradition of yoga discusses the Maya Koshas. These are layers of the self that we train in order to reach bliss or enlightenment. Like a nesting doll, we remove one layer to get to the next one. The first layer to address is Annamaya Kosha which is roughly translated to food body. This is the physical body, the exterior layer, of the self that is necessary to train in order to begin training the more subtle parts of ourselves—like our thoughts, emotions, and energy.

Buddhism describes the body as being the gateway to the mind, "To keep the body in good health is a duty; otherwise we shall not be able to keep our mind strong and clear."

In the Christian faith, the Bible calls our body a temple: "Do you not know that your bodies are temples of the Holy Spirit, who is in you, whom you have received from God? Therefore, honor God with your bodies." — 1 Corinthians 6:19-20.

The Islamic faith considers our bodies to be a gift or a trust from Allah. We should not abuse it or neglect it.

The Jewish faith considers taking care of one's body a mitzvah (commandment). The body is viewed as a channel to one's soul.

CHARACTER POWER TOOLS

Who do we get to become if our body knows strength and balance? If we have a strong, balanced body, we are more capable of using our power tools. Bonus—our power tools also help us build a strong physical body. It's a win-win situation!

Courage

Specifically, we need to have the courage to move more. It often takes courage to start moving, to increase movement, and to commit to moving. Courage is finding the edge that is between doable and challenging—pushing ourselves to do a harder-than-usual workout. Succeeding often nudges us to do something courageous in another part of our life. An example of this may be *Since I pushed through and endured that really hard workout, I feel courageous and confident to have that difficult conversation.*

We build confidence by doing something that challenges us—learning a new movement or physical activity, meeting or exceeding a goal. Some people need courage just to start a movement routine. Some of us need courage to "be imperfect" at an activity. If you tend toward seeking perfection and are reluctant to start something new because of that, try going way in the other direction. Add laughter or singing to your activity. Be silly. Play.

Crawl, walk, run. When we begin our activity, we may only be able to move hard for thirty seconds at a time before we are out of breath. But we did it. We moved. Let's inspire ourselves with encouraging phrases:

- Tomorrow I'll go forty seconds!
- Better and better, one day at a time!

- Never been a better day to be my best!

Simplicity

When we start a movement practice, let's make it simple and doable. We can always add more as time goes on. What movements can we do consistently, even for a short duration initially? How can we incorporate activities that raise our heart rate, strengthen our muscles, and focus on balance and flexibility? Consider Jake's story about getting off the couch and running for ten minutes. Or think of Cole's story about doing push-ups against the bathtub.

Positivity

Consider the benefits that movement adds to our life. Think about the words we use around movement. Are we acknowledging that we are feeling stronger, more in touch with ourselves? Or are we telling ourselves that we are too fat or weak, and will never be able to lift as much as Hank at the gym? Remember that our self-talk affects our movement. The more positive our self-talk, the stronger our body responds. This is an example of a mind-body connection. Jake describes how he used to grind through his workouts, his face outwardly revealing anger. His coach asked him why he was so pissed off whenever he worked out. Jake took a moment and realized his self-talk was, "Come on, you can do better, you worthless piece of shit!" Though our self-talk may be slightly more supportive than Jake's, let's listen to it. If it is negative, we can turn it around and make it positive and encouraging. Let's even try to smile during our movement exercises. Some people may think we are a little loony; they are welcome to think that. Simply smiling will invite positivity into our workout. And we may make a few new friends.

Our society needs to get rid of regarding physical activity as something to dread. Think of the myriad benefits that movement provides us. We have virtually a limitless number of ways to move our bodies. If we don't like to sweat, we can stretch, do tai chi, do certain types of yoga, walk, or dance in our kitchen. We don't have to endure long, grueling sessions of 250 burpees followed by a five-mile run. Unless that is your jam.

Commitment

Let's plan to succeed. Let's decide to move daily. This is a promise to our Self. We can add movement to our daily self-care routine, just like washing our face and brushing our teeth. Whenever we have a moment, let's just move. If we are at home with children during the day, our movement may need to be flexible—push-ups against the bathtub. Some people may want to schedule their workouts in the morning while their partner stays with the kids. A positive aspect of a morning workout routine is that we incorporate the effects of our feel-good neurotransmitters into the rest of our day. As movement becomes a regular habit, you'll notice the confidence and motivation that become part of daily life.

Resilience

A conditioned body is inherently more resilient on all levels of our Self. It helps us become more resistant to environmental changes, illnesses, injuries, depression, and enhances our overall wellbeing.

We can also practice resilience when we experience discomfort or get injured. It may seem easiest to simply stop all movement activities and say, "I just knew this whole physical activity shit wasn't for me!" No. Let's not do that. Instead, we can turn to a different movement, such as yoga or another type of recovery practice. For example, if we injure some part of our lower body, what movements can we do that involves our upper body muscles? We can use this time to let our creative juices flow and tap into the resilience strategy of flexibility.

Awareness

Our body generously provides clues to what is happening inside us. We can witness our body through somatic (body) awareness. This involves tuning into our body, assessing our physical sensations. What sensations are we feeling? Are we experiencing pain or tightness anywhere? Is our physical discomfort related to emotionally feeling tense or anxious? Are we feeling more fatigued today? Are we feeling resistant to moving our body today? Why?

Deep breathing is a tool that lets us observe sensations that we may not otherwise be conscious of. By focusing on breath, we quiet the mind long enough to hear our thoughts, feel our emotions, and experience the sensations of our bodies. Remembering not to judge our thoughts and sensations, we can rely on our breath for awareness during times of stillness and times of movement.

Tuning into our breath helps us gauge the ease and intensity of our physical activity. Are we breathing hard but still able to carry on a conversation? If so, this is moderate-intensity activity. Are we breathing hard but can only say a few words before taking a breath? This is high-intensity activity. You may have heard of high-intensity interval training, known as HIIT. HIIT involves short intervals of high-intensity activity followed by rest periods. The average duration of a HIIT session is ten to thirty minutes. It provides the same health benefits as a moderate-intensity workout that lasts twice as long. So, for those of us who feel short on time during the day, we can do this type of workout. We won't have any trouble being aware of our breath with HIIT.

Using habit awareness, what habits do you currently have around movement? Is movement already scheduled into your day? Think about your present daily activities. Are there any that you'd like to change? Where can you fit movement into your daily life?

Purpose

Does movement fit into why and how you want to live? You are choosing to move daily. What purpose does it serve? Do you really want to live with more strength, energy, positivity, and be more mentally fit?

Our purpose serves as our intention to live a certain way. Though we may not be able to verbalize our purpose yet, we can ask ourselves if we are presenting our best Self to those we love. This is the underlying reason Jake decided to get off the couch and become active. He realized his lack of energy and irritability was not contributing to a high quality of life for him, his wife, or his children. He did not want to live this way or be remembered for these qualities. Without knowing that he was turning the key to unlock his purpose, he knew he needed to work on himself in order to give to those he loved. Flight attendants understand this concept very well, "Please place the oxygen mask over your own mouth and nose before assisting others." If we are functionally and physically unfit for our own life, how can we fully assist others?

HOW CAN I PERSONALLY APPLY MOVEMENT TO MY LIFE RIGHT NOW?

Start anywhere. Pick any activity and decide to do it daily. As we said, the daily practice of movement is more important than the final result. The goal is the habit.

We all have ten-minute chunks of time available in our days to move. Try to get thirty minutes of movement or physical activity per day. It doesn't matter if it is broken up into three ten-minute sessions or you do it all at once. Short bursts of activity each day are a great place to start.

Decide to move throughout your day. Set your phone alarm to stand and do some stretches or a quick set of lunges. Consider starting with a couple of different movements. Make them simple and doable. Do some push-ups and squats. If you can't do a full push-up, start on your knees; if you can only crank out five at first, great! You've made progress. Go for six push-ups next week.

Just decide to move!

- Set up a system for success.
- Schedule your movement times.
- Put it on the calendar.
- Find a workout buddy.
- Include your partner and children in your activities.

For those who are past the starting phase of movement or already have a workout routine, is there a challenge or type of movement that you could train for? How could your current workout routine become more integrated? For example, could you incorporate range-of-motion movements, balance, strength, cardio, recovery, and breath practice? Once physical activity becomes a habit, we can focus on increasing our skills, capacity, and endurance. Think of connecting your training to a deeper part of who you are. How can your training help you build your character power tools? If we associate our training with the many other areas it affects in our self and relationships, we realize the numbers on the scale are simply one measurement among all of the movement benefits.

HOW CAN WE USE MOVEMENT TO HELP STRENGTHEN OUR MARRIAGE?

Healthy behavior can be a fun team sport. Whenever we move or work out with our partner, we work on two growth areas at once: Movement and Connection. During movement activities, we can encourage each other, gently push each other, and practice communicating even during higher intensity activities. We can lovingly hold each other accountable to our healthy lifestyle.

What are your dreams together? Think about future vacations or events you'd like to do. Do you want to hike the Grand Canyon together? Think outside the box for ideas of physical activities to do as a couple. Create activities that have a sense of adventure and excitement. Now that movement has increased our brain's creativity, let's use that creativity.

Regular physical activity can lead to a healthier and more satisfying sex life. Sex itself is physical activity. (It is also an emotional and spiritual activity, as we will address later.) Sex helps deepen our relationship with our partner as well as helps us live longer. What more do we want? The research on the Blue Zones found that eighty percent of people between the ages of sixty-five and one hundred were having sex—yet another reason for us to get moving (Buettner 2012).

Having our own movement practice and working on ourself tells our partner, "I care about you, and I want to be here for you. One reason I am taking care of myself is that I want to bring my best self to you." Keep in mind that you don't have to do every physical activity together. You may not enjoy the same movement activities. But make sure to give and take a little bit. If your partner loves yoga and it's not your favorite thing, decide to do yoga together once a week (or once a month). If you go into the activity with a positive attitude, you will find something you like about it. It also is an example of love in action. Remember to have fun together. You are a couple, strengthening your relationship. Take advantage of the neurotransmitters' mood-elevating effects together. Go enjoy!

IDEAS OF ACTIVITIES TO ENJOY TOGETHER:

- Yoga
- Walking or hiking
- Biking
- Active volunteering
- Adventuring or rock climbing
- Dancing (ballroom or simply in the kitchen)
- Training for a fun themed race (Mud Run, Monster Dash)
- Walking your dog
- Sex
- Skiing or snowshoeing
- Kayaking or canoeing
- Playing golf

- Playing tennis

- Simply scheduling surprise movement date

HOW CAN WE USE MOVEMENT TO HELP STRENGTHEN OUR RELATIONSHIP WITH OUR FAMILY?

With kids, physical activity is about fun and experience. They don't think of movement as a workout. As parents, we want to be a positive part of our children's memories. Children love to move, and they love to spend time with us. Let's go to the park and play with them. When they ask us to play, let's change our default answer to "Yes," even when we don't feel like it. When they ask, "Do you want to play tag with us outside?" We answer, "Yes," even though we would rather stay in our warm house, finishing the latest novel by Vince Flynn. When they ask us to swim with them, we answer, "Oh, in the 52-degree water? Sure!" Usually, by the time we start playing, focusing on the moment, we remember that playing is fun. Even if we are cold.

Though we want our kids to play and create their own movement activities, organized sports have a role as well. Sports teach movement skills that our children can carry through to adulthood. We are fortunate to have a wide offering of organized activities today. They teach our kids how to work hard and work together as a team. The benefits of movement, the team atmosphere, and learning through sports can offer our children life-long benefits. Organized sports can also be a detriment—to our child and to our family. How does the overall sports activity affect our child? Do they generally enjoy it and look forward to the activity? Even if they don't look forward to it, do they seem to enjoy the sport once they start playing? How does the activity affect the dynamic of our family? Our marriage? Our other children? Let's keep in mind that if our child someday becomes an all-star at their chosen sport, it will be because of their internal drive to do so. It will be due to their personal passion. It will not come from us yelling at them from the sidelines or paying thousands of dollars for them to be on the best teams. It will not happen if the stress and busyness tear our family apart. This is an area to use our awareness tool—to periodically check in and assess how each member of our team is doing.

Children don't want to be forced into a physical activity that they don't enjoy doing. If you love to go for a run and your child does not, consider inviting them to go while giving them the option to decline. Leave the door open so they can choose. You may be surprised that after a month, your child decides to join you for the first block of your run. We want our kids to associate physical activity with positive moments.

Schedule movement dates or weekends with your family. Make them fun, goofy, memorable. Do you have multiple children? Give each child their own day to plan a family activity or a one-on-one activity with just Mom or just Dad.

IDEAS OF FAMILY ACTIVITIES TO ENJOY TOGETHER:

- Having a snowball fight
- Building a fort
- Sledding, skiing, or snowshoeing
- Active volunteering
- Playing tag or Hide-and-Seek
- Adventuring or having a scavenger hunt
- Ice skating or inline skating
- Biking and running
- Having a relay race or obstacle course
- Dancing (even to a video game)
- Walking as a family or with your dog
- Kayaking or canoeing
- Swimming
- Playing golf or tennis
- Having a family or neighborhood game

Our kids are always watching and listening to us, even if it doesn't appear so. We model the importance of movement and physical activity as well as the language we use around it. Our children watch us move, they hear us talk about movement and sports, they hear us talk about our body, and they notice how we talk and act when we watch them from the bleachers. So, what are your children seeing and hearing?

SUMMARY:

Physical activity gives us a strong foundation that supplies two-way communication lines between our body and our brain. Daily movement has many benefits. It will help us live longer, more fulfilling lives. It will help us be more physically and mentally fit. We are more apt to fight off infections, disease, and we will grow our brain. Daily movement will help squash that irritability that can creep up on us; it allows us to think more clearly and feel more deeply. We can enjoy a range of new activities with our partner, and we can actively play with our kids! Now that we know how to strengthen our body, let's learn how to fuel it and maintain it. We need high-quality fuel and robust construction materials to keep our foundation strong!

CHAPTER 9
NUTRITION

Having a strong physical body has many benefits. It is our base. Movement is one way to strengthen the body. Movement can't build strong muscles and bones alone, though. Our physical body needs to be made of and fueled by long-lasting materials. High-quality nutrition is needed to support a firm foundation. Nutrition helps maintain our strength for the duration.

Through another lens, we can view movement as our body's output. It is something our body performs or produces. What about the input? What are we putting into our body to develop and maintain its structure—to enable it to move? Are we using high-quality, top-tier fuel to optimize our body's functions? Or are we choosing foods simply because they are cheap or convenient? The food and drinks that pass through our mouth affect every aspect of our body. Movement and nutrition work together to maintain the very foundation of our Self. Let's create and maintain a strong one.

THE DIET INDUSTRY

The diet industry—a $150 billion industry in the United States and Europe—focuses on what and when to eat. Diet plans are based on partial truths related to some part of our health. But they all fall short because they aren't individualized to anyone's personal body or life. Many diets emphasize "good" or "bad" when discussing types of foods, the amount of food, and the timing of meals. Unfortunately, diet plans are created to rely on their system and to make money rather than rely on ourselves. This all-or-nothing mentality may work for the military, but we continue to find that it doesn't work for the general civilian population. We are in the midst of an obesity epidemic. And we are undernourished. Overweight and undernourished? How can that be possible? The Standard American Diet and "empty calories" are a hint.

Similar to fitness center advertisements, diet plans tout a better body image as the result of weight loss. Body image—our thoughts, perceptions, and attitude about our body—should be under our control, not dictated by advertisements or diet plans. What is society's ideal body image anyway? It is elusive on purpose; therefore, we will always be chasing an undefined ideal. "Body image concerns affect girls as young as six years of age. Forty to sixty percent of elementary school girls are concerned about their weight or about becoming fat. This concern endures through life" (Smolak 2011). What is going on here? It's time to flip the script. The National Eating Disorders Association offers two programs that promote positive body image and healthy eating patterns. The Confident Body,

Confident Child program is aimed at children from ages two to six. The Body Project is a group-based support program for high school girls and college-aged women. We are seeing some movement toward accepting healthy bodies of different shapes and sizes, but the movement is slow. Numerous research studies have revealed that the media contributes to the relationship people have with their bodies. Developing media awareness and a better understanding of its influence will help us and our children create healthier relationships with our bodies. Beauty, success, and self-esteem are not determined by thinness. Beauty, success, and self-esteem arise from a confident, healthy, strong Self.

NUTRITION IN A NUTSHELL

We are going to focus on why and how we eat—exploring our relationship with food. We will learn to listen to our body signals. We aren't going to recommend a regimented diet plan or specific foods. Our bodies simply are not one-size-fits-all. The type and amount of food that a 250-pound male endurance athlete needs are very different than what a 120-pound sedentary female needs to fuel their body. We want you to get to know your individual body. We will focus on how to become aware of the best fuels to optimize the function of our body.

At its core, nutrition is the study of how our body uses the nutrients in food and the relationship between diet, health, and disease. Nutrients are tiny substances in food that every part of our body needs for health, growth, and life. Nutrients include proteins, vitamins, minerals, water, and healthy carbohydrates and fats.

Nutrient-dense foods contain a high amount of nutrients and are low in calories. They contain healthy fats and little to no added sugar and salt. Salmon, kale, and broccoli are only a few examples of the many nutrient-dense foods.

Energy-rich and nutrient-poor foods are high in calories (energy) and provide very few nutrients. This is where the term "empty calories" comes from. Research suggests that the Standard American Diet is high in energy-rich, nutrient-poor foods (eatrightpro.org 2016). We want to minimize eating foods such as these—foods that don't help our body, and in high amounts, hurt our body.

Amidst the years of trendy diets, one piece of research has remained the same—nutrient-dense food choices positively affect all aspects of our health in the short- and long-term. Energy-rich and nutrient-poor food choices negatively affect our health in the short- and long-term.

SO WHY IS HEALTHY NUTRITION REALLY IMPORTANT?

You may have heard the phrase "Food is medicine." How and what we eat can make us sick, or it can keep us healthy and prevent disease. And what is the definition of medicine? Merriam-Webster defines medicine as "a substance or preparation used in treating disease; something that affects well-being" (Merriam-Webster 2021). Sound vaguely similar?

Food as medicine—now that's an inexpensive, easy-to-use treatment compared to swallowing a pill or giving ourselves an insulin injection! And with fewer side effects.

What does healthy nutrition really do? The tiniest components of our body are our cells. They need specific nutrients found in food. If we supply those nutrients to our body through the foods we eat, our cells function as they should. Our body has billions of cells that have a number of functions. We have brain cells that differ from muscle cells that differ from lung cells. They all need nutrients to function in these different ways to keep our body healthy and prevent disease. If we don't regularly provide our body with the needed nutrients, we are essentially telling our cells, "You are not that important. Go ahead and do what you want—shut down, get sick, divide yourselves, whatever." Breast Cancer.org reports that nutrition is partly responsible for 30% to 40% of breast cancer. Since nutrients are needed for our cells to function in a healthy manner, and cancer is defined by cells that are not functioning as they should, it is fairly easy to see a connection between poor nutrition and diseases such as cancer.

We know that nutrients are essential for growth and the maintenance of life, but can one nutrient really impact our body? Let's look at the nutrient called magnesium. Magnesium is needed for healthy cells in many different body systems. Magnesium is needed for controlling our blood sugar, cholesterol, and blood pressure; for maintaining healthy bones, nerves, muscles, and blood vessels; and for supporting our immune system. One nutrient, a mineral typically found in the soil, profoundly affects our health and wellness. What if we said, "I am not going to eat magnesium-containing foods because I don't like the way they taste?" Knowing all of the benefits magnesium provides our body, we reply, "Self, not everything that passes our lips has to give us a food buzz! We are eating to support and maintain all the connections in this body." (As a note, a variety of foods contain magnesium, so it would be highly unusual to dislike all magnesium-containing foods. Plus, dark chocolate happens to be a good source of magnesium!)

The perks of healthy nutrition go beyond our own physical body. The associated behaviors and traditions around nutrition affect the strength and mental health of our family. In his book The Power of Full Engagement, author Jim Loehr said, "Every time we participate in a ritual, we express our beliefs. Families who sit down together for dinner are saying without words that shared time together is important" (Loehr 2003). As an aside to Jim's quote, the meal doesn't just have to be dinner. It can be any meal. If we add just one more meal together with our family during the week, it increases the following benefits:

- Connection and bonding time which encourages open conversation
- Improved, healthier food choices, food variety, and lower soda consumption among children
- Lower rates of obesity for children and adults
- Lower rates of substance abuse and pregnancy in teens

The key to family meals is to make them enjoyable occasions. Respect everyone's voice. Our family meals are rituals that will become etched in our children's memories.

NUTRITION AND PHYSICAL ACTIVITY

What about nutrition as it relates to movement and physical activity? How does nutrition affect our stamina, our recovery, or even our motivation to get off the couch? Fortunately, a lot of research has been done about the relationship between nutrition and physical activity. Healthy nutrition is now viewed as one of the most important parts of fitness programs. When we are physically active, our body often requires more consistent, efficient fuel. Healthy food gives our body the energy that is needed for physical activity. It can further help us reach our fitness goals, reduce the risk of injury, and help us recover more quickly after physical activity. The type and amount of foods we eat will depend on our unique body as well as the amount and intensity of our activity. If we are moving daily and get in about 150 minutes of physical activity within a week, we don't need to increase our calorie intake. For those of us who engage in high-intensity workouts or long endurance activities, our nutritional needs will be different. Regardless of where we are on the activity scale, we are better off filling our tanks with high-quality fuel in the form of nutrient-dense foods. Nutrient-dense foods—also called superfoods—have a naturally high concentration of vitamins, minerals, and powerful cell-defenders known as antioxidants. Antioxidants reduce inflammation in our body. They help protect us from illnesses and diseases. Remember how our cells take in the nutrients that they need from the food we eat? Think of antioxidants as armor for our cells, protecting them from free radical damage. (Dark chocolate happens to be an antioxidant as well. Are you noticing a theme here?)

Though our bodies differ, we each need to have balanced nutrition. We need to eat a variety of foods to make sure we are getting adequate nutrients, in addition to vitamins and minerals. The ratio of nutrients needed for our individual body may vary, but in general, we need:

- Protein. Our body needs protein to maintain and repair muscles. Protein reduces muscle soreness.

- Carbohydrates. Our body needs carbohydrates to give us energy and help us perform at our best. We can think of carbohydrates as the key fuel for our brain and muscles during exercise. Choose whole food carbohydrates such as vegetables, fruits, and whole grains like brown rice. They contain essential nutrients and fiber to provide us with lasting energy. Our body will break down the whole carb food into usable energy.

- Fat. Our body needs a small but consistent amount of healthy fats for a variety of functions. It protects our organs, helps with cell growth, keeps our blood pressure and cholesterol under control, and helps our body absorb nutrients. Unsaturated fats are the healthy kind. These include fats from plants, such as avocados, nuts, seeds, plant oils; and fish, such as salmon, tuna, or herring.

- Water. Our body needs water simply to maintain itself every day. Our body loses water simply by breathing. During physical activity, our increased body temperature and sweat cause us to lose even more water. Not surprisingly, our body performs its best and recovers more quickly when we drink enough water. As a society, we are generally mildly dehydrated (low on water). This can cause us to be tired or crabby, and have brain fog or headaches. Even mild dehydration can reduce our strength and endurance when we are moving.

Water is best for our body, even when exercising. And it is cheap. We don't need sports drinks unless we are extremely active and engaging in endurance exercise for more than an hour. Sports drinks contain a type of sugar called glucose that our cells can use immediately. They also contain electrolytes such as sodium (salt) to replace any that was lost during sweating. Other chemicals are often added as well. If you or your kids exercise in a way that requires sports drinks, consider making your own. Just crush some fresh fruit into a puree, add a pinch of salt, and fill the remainder of the container with water. Homemade sports drinks only use simple ingredients without added chemicals.

Energy drinks, on the other hand, are not sports drinks. They are not designed to replace electrolytes lost during physical activity. Many are high in sugar and chemicals, and they contain a potentially dangerous amount of stimulants, such as caffeine and taurine. Energy drinks are not recommended for children. They will not help your child jump higher, run faster, or aim straighter. Instead, they can cause dangerously high heart rates, extreme hyperactivity, seizures, and even a stroke in children. If your children are thirsty, toss them a bottle of water.

NUTRITION AND OUR GUT MICROBIOME

The gut microbiome—what a mouthful! The gut, as we are using it here, consists of our stomach and intestines. Billions of bacteria, viruses, fungi, and other micro-sized organisms live in our gut. This generally happy community of microbes is called our gut microbiome. It plays a large role in digesting the food we eat, and as researchers are finding, it is involved in a number of other processes that occur in our body.

Most of the gut microbes are good for our body, yet some can be harmful. The beneficial microbes multiply so often that they keep the potentially harmful microbes in check. This balance allows the microbes to exist together without problems. But if something disturbs the balance—such as an illness, poor nutrition, prolonged use of antibiotics, or stress—the normal microbial interactions get out of whack. Our body becomes more susceptible to inflammation and chronic diseases.

Research continues to shine a light on the microbiome and its importance to our overall health. It plays a role in so many of our body functions that it is becoming known as its own organ—our body's second brain. Since nutrition has such an effect on the microbiome, we want to touch on some of this so-called organ's health-promoting functions.

- It strengthens our immune system, increasing our body's ability to prevent and fight illnesses and diseases.

- It helps our body absorb and use the nutrients from the foods we eat.

- It reduces inflammation throughout our body and regulates our blood sugar.

- It affects our mood and behavior. Depression, anxiety, and neurodegenerative diseases (Alzheimer's disease, Parkinson's disease, Multiple Sclerosis) can all be positively affected by a healthy gut microbiome.

An interesting aspect of the microbiome is that it is ever-changing. The type and number of microbes can vary daily, weekly, or monthly depending on factors that we can control—our food choices, exercise, medicines, and how much water we drink. In fact, these factors can impact our gut microbes within twenty-four hours.

A healthy gut microbiome needs a variety of foods to maintain the diversity of microbes. We can provide nutrients to the good microbes to strengthen them. Foods that feed the good microbes include:

- Whole foods (fruits, vegetables, seeds, nuts, beans, whole grains) that are naturally high in fiber. The fiber in whole foods is the nutrient that feeds the good bacteria.

- Polyphenols which are found in fruits, tea, dark chocolate, red wine

- Prebiotic fibers found in onions, garlic, asparagus, bananas
- Probiotics (live bacteria) found in fermented foods such as yogurt, kefir, pickles, kombucha, sauerkraut

So, let's remember that when choosing the foods we put in our mouth, we are feeding the billions of microbes as well. The more diverse our foods, the more diverse the microbes. Eating a variety of foods is healthy for our gut as well as our entire body.

NUTRITION AND BRAIN HEALTH

Nutrition is essential for a well-functioning brain. It helps us think and process information more clearly. The neurotransmitter serotonin that helps regulate our mood, sleep, and appetite is mainly produced in our gut. Ninety-five percent of this chemical—a brain chemical—is produced in the gut! Not surprisingly, the function of serotonin is influenced by the health of our gut microbiome. Healthy nutrition has been shown to improve mental health problems such as depression, bipolar disorder, schizophrenia, and ADHD. It also works with physical activity to reduce the risk of Alzheimer's disease.

The long-living people in the Blue zones eat foods consistent with those associated with the Mediterranean diet. Mediterranean diet foods include fruits, vegetables, legumes, whole grains, nuts, olive oil, and a balance of red meat, dairy products, and saturated fats. The foods are heart-healthy and flavorful—and are promoted by both western and eastern medicine. What's more is this type of nutrition is associated with less inflammation in the brain and body, positive benefits to the gut microbiome, and overall long-term good health.

HIGHLY REFINED, PROCESSED FOODS. WHAT'S THE DEAL?

Processed food is any food that has undergone a change from its natural state. This includes washing, cleaning, cooking, freezing, canning, chopping, etc. Most of the food we find in our grocery stores falls under that definition. Minimal processing doesn't greatly affect the food's nutrient content. However, the nutrient content in highly processed foods can be destroyed or removed. Even moderately processed foods involve peeling the outer layer of fruits, vegetables, and whole grains. Heating and drying foods can further strip them of their vitamins and minerals. Sometimes food manufacturers are able to add some of the lost nutrients back into the food, calling the foods fortified, but the full benefit of the whole food has been lost. Highly refined, processed foods are the products to which people often refer when talking about unhealthy American foods. The foods are packaged in a shelf-stable way and contain added sugar, salt, and fat. Artificial colors, flavors, and preservatives are also added. Unfortunately, these food additives are not tested on how they react with our gut microbiome. Highly refined, processed foods are linked to an increase in obesity, diabetes, and heart disease. A number of studies are being done to explore the connection between highly processed foods and inflammation in the body. The results suggest that people reduce their risk of inflammatory diseases if they reduce their intake of highly processed foods in their diets. Essentially, processed foods are not designed to enhance our well-being. They are designed to sell and to make money. Highly processed foods are often chemically engineered to be hyperpalatable (excessively pleasing to our tastebuds). Whole foods, such as foods found in nature, are flavorful. However, highly processed foods that contain a calculated amount of fat, sugar, and salt create an intensely pleasurable flavor. These foods light up the reward center in our brain on MRI scans. They overpower mechanisms in our brain that signal when we've had enough to eat.

In other words, our brain creates a memory of the intense pleasure related to consuming a highly processed food, such as Cheetos®. Our memory of such intense pleasure makes us crave Cheetos®. We overeat the food because our pause-signals aren't working. Thus, we are surprised to discover an empty bag of Cheetos® on our lap, our fingers full of orange dust. The next time we are at the grocery store and see Cheetos® on the shelf, our brain remembers the intense pleasure. Just like Pavlov's dogs, we start to salivate, and the cycle starts all over again.

As we continue our journey to evaluate nutrition and how specific foods affect us, let's pay attention to highly processed foods. Look at the ratio of calories to nutrients on the package. The higher the ratio of calories to nutrients, the unhealthier the food. We can practice using our Awareness power tool:

- How do we feel immediately after eating a highly processed food?

- Do we eat the recommended serving size?

- How do we feel an hour after eating the food?

- How is our stamina and strength during physical activity? Do we see a connection between how we feel and how we perform?

OUR RELATIONSHIP WITH FOOD

Jake describes his relationship with food as somewhat of a roller coaster. As a young adult, he felt that he could eat whatever and whenever he wanted. He could also practically drink his weight in calories—and we are not talking about soda. Jake didn't pay attention to how food affected him. He physically trained for or played hockey every day, so his weight wasn't affected. Once Jake transitioned into a more sedentary line of work, he thought he could just do a major ass-kicking workout to undo the massive quantities of food he put in his mouth. As you may recall, Jake was told that he looked angry or pissed off whenever he worked out. He was trying to undo a six-pack of beer and a large pizza. We'd look pissed too! Jake now says that he feels the impact of his food choices more acutely. He is more in tune with his body and its sensations. He uses these sensations as learning tools on how best to fuel his body. He has been amazed at not only the physical impacts his food choices have made on his body but also the emotional impacts, including his mood and energy.

Jake is married with two children and, like many of us, has a lot going on in his life. The challenge around nutrition has centered around time. Living full, busy lives, his family found it nearly essential to choose fast, easy foods. This seemed to work fine until a life-altering nutritional diagnosis occurred in their family. One of Jake's children was diagnosed with a GI condition known as ulcerative colitis. This changed the family's perspective on diet and nourishment. With the goal of improving the whole family's health and nutrition, they decided to practice simplicity to accommodate their busy schedules and more complex health needs. They became acutely aware of the need for individualization of food and the need to focus on their family mealtimes. Jake says that their meals don't have to be fancy, but simple foods work for them and give them time to enjoy each other.

What is your relationship to food, to mealtimes? What are your habits around the foods you routinely eat, food preparation, grocery shopping? What is your general eating schedule? How about water and hydration? Alcohol? Finally, where do you eat—at the table, in your car, in front of the TV? When we become aware of our relationship with food, we can form a baseline. What are we currently doing that we want to continue? What could we improve on or do differently?

MINDFUL EATING

It is becoming the norm to eat quickly and mindlessly. We are so busy and feel the need to rush to our next activity. This, in addition to our generation's low-grade fatigue and mind-numbing carpools, leads to eating highly processed, flavorful foods—especially foods that give us a burst of sugar and dopamine. Hello, Oreos®! Our body can use the calories from such foods for energy. Until the sugar crash. However, our cells can't find nutrients in these foods to keep healthy. These packaged empty-calorie foods are convenient, and they taste good. And, yes, we like to eat them from time to time. It's when we make them part of our daily nutrition habit that our health starts to suffer.

When we slow down and become aware while we eat, we reduce our stress, make better choices, and help our body digest. Slower, mindful eating allows our body to absorb nutrients more easily from the foods we eat. When we are physically or emotionally distracted, our brain perceives these distractions as stress. As we know from the fight-or-flight response, digestion and metabolism are reduced. The digestive process is simply not a priority when our body is in the red zone.

How can we practice mindful eating?

- Before eating, assess if you are physically hungry. Is your stomach growling? Are you low on energy? Are we actually thirsty instead of hungry?

- Sit down at a table for meals.

- Eliminate distractions such as phones, TV, or other devices. Just set them aside.

- Keep the environment relatively calm. Consider playing relaxing or instrumental music.

- Focus on the smell, taste, and texture of your food.

- Think about how the nutrients are going to affect your body.

- What signals does your body send when it has had enough to eat?

We don't have to be a member of the "Clean Plate Club." Regardless of what our parents said, the health of the children in Africa will not be affected by the amount of food left on our plate. It will take awareness and discipline to re-think how and why we eat.

Food as fuel—what a healthy concept to establish with our kids! We can use visualization games as early examples of mindful eating with our children:

- When the kids are eating a healthy food, have them picture the food as they swallow it.

- The food contains tiny superheroes called nutrients. Can they imagine the little superheroes breaking away from the food they just swallowed and entering the cells in their body?

- As a superhero enters the cell, the cell's light turns on, and the cell begins to grow. Now, do they notice that the bright cell looks stronger?

- Wait, is the cell flexing its teeny muscles and giving us a high-five?

Visualization games help foster healthier eating in children. Maybe as a child, you were encouraged to eat spinach to develop muscles like Popeye. What visualization stories can you put together that would inspire your kids? The sillier, the better.

HOW IS NUTRITION REFLECTED IN TRADITIONS?

Food and nutritional habits continue to be basic parts of many cultures and traditions. Food has played a large role in celebrations and ceremonies, such as during holidays or religious feasts. It has symbolized love. Certain religious requirements, such as fasting and avoiding pork, have been practiced for thousands of years as a form of honor and discipline. Humans have also used food and nutritional habits to treat illnesses and maintain their health. Among the world's old and new traditions that center on food, do any of them focus on how our food habits will make us look in a swimming suit?

CHARACTER POWER TOOLS

Who do we get to become if our body is nutritionally healthy? When we are nutritionally healthy, we are more capable of using our power tools. Our power tools will also help us in our journey to become more nutritionally healthy.

Courage

As we know, it takes courage to make any change and to stick with it. Eating with awareness or in a mindful manner most likely will be a change. It may seem slow and cumbersome until it becomes a newly created habit. Our kids may grumble. We may grumble. Yet, we can go into the change expecting that. Remember that courage is the choice to do something uncomfortable.

It takes courage to stand our ground when eating with friends or engaged in foodie activities that we've participated in for years. What if our friends host an annual party that includes foods commonly found at the State Fair? We have a choice. Since no foods are off-limits to us and we know how our own body responds, we may decide to imbibe in a gyro followed by a deep-fried Twinkie® and a snack-size, deep-fried Snickers®. We may even decide to wash all of this down with a glass of milk straight from a cow's udder. If that is the case, we need to give ourselves grace and permission to enjoy these foods during this special occasion. On the other hand, if we decide that eating those foods isn't worth the effect they will have on our body, we can courageously explain this to our friends. We don't mean to end a tradition; we can continue such a celebration, and we might add some foods to it. We can consider preparing or bringing some food to the party that we know helps our body feel stronger and offer to share it with the group. Who knows—maybe cucumbers and hummus will be a great accompaniment to the deep-fried feast.

We don't want to become complacent or avoid paying attention to our nutrition. We want to be conscious and deliberate. We need courage to fuel ourselves in ways that are meaningful to us and our journey. The common consumption of the Standard American Diet is easy to fall into. It is hyper-convenient. Courage to choose the uncommon will keep our foundation strong.

Simplicity

Nutrition as a concept can be quite complex. Heck, the study of nutrition is a four-year college degree! When we focus on our relationship with our family as well as our relationship with food, what can we do that is simple and meaningful? We may need to take a step back and think about what brings us joy. Where again do we find meaning? An elaborate dinner consisting of Grandma's whole roasted turkey, mashed potatoes, and salad followed by a homemade apple pie may be meaningful to us. But is the four-hour prep simple or realistic after a full day of work? Let's listen to our self-talk. Is it really true that the only good meals should look like those made by our grandmother? Healthy nutrition can be simple.

- Consider looking online for recipes that are designed to be simple and healthy, and used for busy families.

- Consider serving simple foods such as baked chicken breasts, a baked potato, and microwave-steamed vegetables. Add spices or sauces that you have in your refrigerator.

- Consider having a meal-prep day once a week. Assemble, cook, or bake several meals. Refrigerate or freeze them to eat later in the week.

- Consider gathering a group of several friends. Ask them each to make their favorite main dish. Instead of only making a serving size for their family, have them make enough so each friend will have a family serving to take home.

- Consider making certain meals on designated days. Taco Tuesday—everyone knows what to expect for dinners on Tuesdays. We always know what ingredients we need in the house. It's a simple meal to prep and serve.

When it comes to simplicity and nutrition, changes are more likely to stick when we make one meaningful change at a time. An example may be to pack some healthy snacks to eat in the car one day a week to replace a fast-food stop. Or drink a glass of water to replace one can of soda (regular or diet). Make one change until the change becomes routine or a habit. Once it is routine, make another meaningful change. Simplicity will allow us to apply our limited energy to what we've decided is most valuable to us.

Positivity

What are the possibilities we want to experience related to nutrition? When we create changes, our brains respond better when we work toward something (include a vegetable with evening meals) rather than against something (avoid all desserts). The positive perspective encourages our brains to look for opportunities—what interesting new vegetables could we try this week? When we focus on what we need to avoid, we respond to a feeling of scarcity. Our options are narrowed, and we end up fixating on what we can't have. It is not enjoyable and not a sustainable way of creating a healthy relationship with food.

How is our language around food? Are there "good" foods and "bad" foods? A healthy relationship with food entails being aware of the foods that strengthen or energize us and which foods do the opposite. Such foods will be different for different people. With that in mind, consider nixing the good food/bad food language since it implies judgment. This is an opportunity to change the conversation in our heads and in our homes. Look for aspects that are positive around food. "That broccoli is such a beautiful color of green!" or "I love the smell of popcorn when we make it on the stove."

In a similar vein, what is our language about the human body? Do we call an overweight person fat, gross, or disgusting? Do we look in the mirror and say similar things about ourselves? How can we reframe language about bodies so that it is positive and doesn't involve judgment? Our coworker Carol may be overweight, but she is strong, energetic, and wickedly smart. Is it our place to judge her regarding her weight or appearance? If we call ourselves a fat slob after eating a particularly delicious birthday meal, how is that moving us forward in a positive manner? What is that teaching our children?

Again, we want to practice positivity during our family mealtimes. We can create a safe, upbeat environment, so mealtimes are about more than just the food. Mealtimes can be an opportunity to teach, to listen, and to deepen trust and relationships. They can be times to laugh. Family meals can be thought of as nourishment for both the body and soul.

Commitment

Commitment is an active dedication to our nutritional goals. Let's associate our goal with a new healthy habit instead of focusing on one final result, such as weight loss. Our habit becomes the goal. We are committed to make this a habit!

We want to commit to our nutritional goals without being overly strict to the point of inflexibility. When we are inflexible, we allow the circumstances that we are trying to control to consume our thoughts. Inflexibility—an all-or-nothing way of thinking—is associated with higher rates of anxiety and depression. It's also associated with goals that are unsustainable. Swearing off "bad" foods or ways of eating is not healthy or realistic. We want to commit to goals that we can maintain. Consider following these 80/20 rules.

- If you choose to eat certain foods that you've found strengthen you, eat those foods 80% of the time. Allow yourself to enjoy other foods 20% of the time.

- Eat until you are 80% full. Our brain takes 20 minutes to catch up to the physical state of our stomach. In addition, eating until we are 80% full rather than stuffed helps us become more mindful of our eating patterns.

So, let's stay focused on our daily habits. Flexibility will help us enjoy and endure the process. Once we make the commitment to healthy nutrition, we make a conscious decision that it is meaningful and is worth the effort.

Resilience

When we fuel our body with the foods it needs for strength, we also increase our stamina—the energy we need to become more resilient. In the physical sense of resilience, the gut microbiome's power can't be overstated. Our body becomes more resilient to illness and disease. Our entire family will have fewer sick days during the year.

If you've tried diets in the past and not stuck with them, you may think your resilience power tool is weak. It's not your resilience. Most diet plans are not sustainable. About two-thirds of all people who "diet" regain the weight they've lost. This is yet another reason to shift our focus away from strict dietary plans, new diet trends, and diets that focus on body image. If we want to lose weight and keep it off, we need to adopt new behaviors—and create new habits! Slow and steady weight loss benefits our whole body, and it is sustainable. Sudden, extreme weight loss can put our body into the unhealthy red zone. Changes that last are best done by tweaking one to two things at a time, opting for choices that provide personal value and meaning. Not a diet brand.

As with any new practice, we are going to make some mistakes. Let's be compassionate with ourselves when this does occur. We are not failures for making mistakes. We are learning what works and what doesn't work for us. We just continue back on our journey—with resilience.

Awareness

Nutrition is intimately associated with awareness. What triggers us to eat? What eating environments do we cultivate? What thoughts and language do we use around food? We have so many opportunities to practice awareness when it comes to nutrition.

Awareness is essential in assessing how various foods impact us—physically, mentally, and emotionally. What signals is our body giving us? Are we physically hungry, or could that feeling be thirst? Could it be boredom? Anxiety?

Do we notice how specific foods or meal patterns affect our partner or children?

How can we focus on being truly mindful or aware of our food in the moment? Can we see it, smell it, feel it, taste it, or hear it as we chew?

How can we practice awareness at mealtimes?

Purpose

How can we connect our relationship with food to our purpose? If our purpose is caring for infants in a Neonatal

Intensive Care Unit, how are we fueling our body to give us the strength and endurance needed to provide such care? If our purpose is to be a positive role model for our children, how are we fueling our body to be such an example? If our partner and children are a big part of our purpose, are we fueling our body to remain healthy, playful, and active for a long life ahead of us? If we can visualize ourselves in the future, let's fuel ourselves to get there.

HOW CAN I PERSONALLY APPLY NUTRITION TO MY LIFE RIGHT NOW?

Where are you already making good choices, and where can you make a change? Set small action steps toward your change goal. The smaller, the better. With small steps, we can see results more quickly and tweak any actions if necessary. Consider creating action steps that apply to one of your nutrition goals. Example: For my goal of eating a leafy green at every dinner, I need to take the action step of going to the farmer's market on Monday and Thursday to buy fresh greens.

Assess your current eating habits during the next week. You'll need to use paper or your journal for this activity.

- Before you eat:

    - Are you physically hungry? How do you know? Could you be feeling bored, excited, nervous, sad, or thirsty?

    - Where are you eating? Are you sitting at a table? Standing at the counter? Eating in your car?

- As you are eating:

  - What are you doing while you are eating? Watching TV? Catching up on work, e-mail, the news, or social media?

  - Are you eating with anybody?

  - Are you noticing different aspects of your food? How does it look? Smell? Taste?

  - Are you eating slowly or quickly? Do you feel rushed?

  - What are the portion sizes of the foods you are eating? How full was your plate?

  - If you are eating different foods, is there a ratio of vegetables and fruits to the rest of the foods?

  - Are you drinking anything? What is it?

- After you finish eating:

  - How did you physically feel after you ate? Were you overly full, or could you have eaten more?

  - Did you feel energized right after you ate? How about an hour after you finished eating?

  - Did you feel tired or sluggish after you ate?

  - Are you able to figure out how a specific food affected you? Also, consider the quantity of food and how quickly you ate it.

HOW CAN WE USE NUTRITION TO HELP STRENGTHEN OUR MARRIAGE?

Discuss nutrition and possible changes you'd like to make regarding nutrition with each other. Keep it an ongoing conversation. What barriers do you predict with your nutrition changes? Will it affect your social lives? Will it require more planning, more time? Healthy nutrition changes mean longer and happier lives together. Just as you would individually, make small, simple changes together as a couple. Don't suddenly opt for a vegan, 18-hour per day fasting program. Nothing can cause marital tension quicker than two grumpy, hangry people.

Encourage each other to keep progressing with your nutrition goals. It's easy to fall back into old habits or patterns without someone there to encourage you. Remember that each of you has a different body. Try to support each other, but not necessarily mimic each other's exact habits. If your partner wants dessert, you don't have to help them eat it or outwardly judge them for choosing it. Be a cheerleader for each other. We've got this!

Examples of actions to do with your partner related to food and nutrition:

- Go on a picnic. It is easier to pack a healthy picnic basket than going to a restaurant. Be creative. During inclement weather, consider making a picnic in a private area of your house.

- Cook healthy meals together. Make it fun. Enjoy a glass of wine, tea, or sparkling water while you interact.

- Take a cooking class together, even if it is online. So many options are available right now. You can take an online class with a chef from Italy or France. Ciao! Oui!

- Taste your way through your local farmer's market. Hold hands and enjoy the walk while you peruse the beans and collard greens.

- Shop for your food at the grocery store together. We know this is taking your date night to another level. However, it can be quality time you have together.

HOW CAN WE USE NUTRITION TO HELP STRENGTHEN OUR RELATIONSHIP WITH OUR FAMILY?

First of all, consider letting your family know how much it means to you to spend time with them during meals. Let them know you love them. Nutrition plays a large role in our children's lifestyle, wellbeing, growth, and development. Family meals provide nurturing and structure that children so strongly desire.

But how do we institute positive mealtimes that include trying new foods? Registered Dietitian Ellyn Satter so eloquently describes the roles and responsibilities of parents and children regarding the subject of eating. She says that "the key parenting responsibilities include providing healthy choices and preparing the food, providing regular meals and snacks, and modeling positive language and behavior around food and mealtimes. Children then are responsible for whether or not they eat the provided foods and how much they consume" (Satter 2019).

As adults, we think of trying a new food as simply taking a bite and deciding whether or not we like the taste and texture. Sometimes we decide this before we even swallow. For children, trying foods begins several steps before they actually put the food into their mouth. It may begin with grocery shopping, helping to identify the food then putting it into the cart. At home, the process may continue with helping prepare the food, smelling, and touching it. They may even play with it at this time. Once the food is prepared, they may want to touch or play with it again, especially if the texture has changed as a result of cooking it. They may smell it or even lick it. Are they at the point yet where they will taste it or put it in their mouth and chew it? That depends on each child.

Think about what makes family mealtimes meaningful or fun for you and your family. Is it realistic to think the only nice mealtime is when the children are sitting quietly in their seats, not squirming? Or they finish all of the food on their plate— followed by, "Thank you for the meal, Mom and Dad. It was truly delicious and so nourishing to our bodies." Not at your house? Consider having a family discussion about mealtimes. Let each family member verbalize their opinion about what makes mealtimes enjoyable or what they would like to change.

Examples of activities to do with your family related to food, nutrition, mealtimes:

- Let little Bobby choose a day to be "in charge" of the family meal. He can choose foods from a healthy framework you provide, add the ingredients to the grocery list, help shop for them, and help prepare the meal. If Bobby voices something he'd like to do to make the meal more meaningful, consider getting the family on board to do it. You may find that Bobby's creative idea of eating like a dog—without using your hands—can be quite an interesting experience.

- Use visualization or art to begin to teach children about nutrition. Can you create a story about bugs in our tummy to explain our gut microbiome? Consider using Play-Doh or clay to make a gut microbiome, using a variety of fun colors to make the bugs. Maybe create some healthy "food" to feed the good bugs.

- Create experiments with food in the kitchen. Let them create their own experiments. What happens if they mix flour, oil, cinnamon, soy sauce, and sparkling water? What does it look like? Can they feel it with their hands? Do they dare taste it?

- Try the raisin sensory experiment together. Put a raisin in front of you. Explore it without judgment.

  - Sight: Look at the raisin on the table. Put it in the palm of your hand. What does it look like? Explore it in detail as if you've never seen it before. What is its shape? What is its color? Is it shiny?

- Touch: Now, move it around in your hand. How does it feel? Is it warm or cold? Is it heavy or light? Is it dry? Is it sticky? Does it leave any residue on your hand? Touch it with one finger. Now grasp it with your thumb and finger. Notice the texture. If you squeeze it, is it squishy?

- Smell: Bring the raisin to your nose and smell it. What does it smell like? How long do you smell it after removing it from under your nose?

- Hearing: Have you ever tried to hear a food before? Put the raisin next to your ear. Move the raisin back and forth between your fingers. Do you hear anything?

- Taste: While holding it between your fingers, place the raisin on the front of your tongue. What do you taste? Move the raisin to the middle, then the side of your tongue. Do you notice any difference in taste? Do you notice an increase in the flow of saliva? Do you have the desire to chew?

- Start to chew. Did you hear anything with your first bite? Did the taste or texture change? Notice how the sound, taste, and texture change while you continue to chew it slowly. Chew it really well before swallowing. As you swallow, do you still feel it? Do you still taste it? How long do you taste it after you've swallowed it?

SUMMARY:

Nutrition consists of nourishing our body, providing the needed nutrients for every cell in our body to function well. Yet, it is more. It is about awareness, relationships, flexibility, and balance. It is about health and strength. We want to become aware of how particular foods affect our body. Does the food strengthen us, give us more stamina, keep us healthy? Or does the food cause us to feel weak, bloated, initially buzzed then tired, or make us sick? Since individual bodies are about as unique as fingerprints, we need to listen to and make decisions for our own body for it to be a strong base.

Nutrition involves relationships—with food itself and with our partner, family, and friends. Nutrition is a bonding experience with our loved ones. It has been for thousands of years.

Flexibility in nutrition allows us to sustain generally healthy patterns while giving ourselves the grace to enjoy the not-so-healthy occasions. We are all anticipating a long journey and want to avoid the rigidity associated with "good" and "bad" foods.

Balanced nutrition means consuming different foods that offer a variety of nutrients. It also means synchronizing our nutrition with our individual needs and activities. Balance is also important for our daily lives and our relationships—the need to balance family mealtimes with other appointments or activities.

If our awareness, relationships, flexibility, or balance is off, our nutrition can suffer. As a result, our health will be affected. In various spiritual traditions, food is described as life we bring into the body. What kind of life are we inviting into our body and homes?

SECTION III

THE MIND SELF

Our mind is the control center of our Self. We now know that this powerhouse doesn't work alone. It requires healthy nutrition and physical activity to function at its best.

Like the last section, we will explore our Mind Self in two parts. First, we will look at discipline. Discipline creates a more focused and purposeful life. We will learn to live deliberately—we will have more energy and fewer temptations. Our disciplines will have deep meaning; and for that reason, they will persevere.

Second, we will examine our mindsets. These include our beliefs. We actually formed our mindsets and beliefs at a young age. We've just added to them as we've matured. Many of our beliefs were imparted on us from our parents, teachers, and coaches. We simply solidified them and stored them away in our brain. Our mindset and beliefs shape our reality. Maybe we should explore them? Anticipate some surprises lurking around that brain of ours.

A healthy, well-examined mind. Let's get started.

CHAPTER 10
DISCIPLINE

Purpose provides meaning and guidance in our day-to-day lives. Discipline is our commitment to a plan of actions that aligns with our purpose. If we asked one hundred people what discipline meant to them, we would receive virtually as many different answers as we had people. Discipline seems to invoke strong opinions as to its meaning and application. Does it mean a set of rules? Punishment? Obedience? Commitment? Compliance? Rigidity? Routine? Dedication? Delay of instant gratification? Standards required to avoid punishment? As with most words that insight various opinions, exploring the word's source can help us narrow down the definition. Discipline originates from the Latin word disciplina, which means "instruction and training." The root word is discere, meaning "to learn." How on earth did we confuse discipline with punishment? Many adults don't recall meaningful, deep teaching and learning as a result of disciplinary actions when they were young. They do remember trying to avoid being disciplined as it was more associated with discomfort, anxiety, and embarrassment. So, let's try to absorb a more positive usage of discipline.

We are going to regard discipline as a deliberate practice of thoughts and actions that aligns with our greater purpose. Discipline is having a really good, consistent plan but modifying the plan if needed. For example, we are disciplined to fuel our body with nutritious foods. We have routinely consumed a glass of milk each day after our workouts over the years. We recently began to notice milk has been causing some stomach issues. Though milk has been part of our routine to fuel our body, we need to eliminate it; we need to modify our plan. Our discipline of fueling our body will remain. The plan will just look a little different.

We are also going to look at discipline in the context of doing—to consistently learn, train, and develop self-control to do what we know is right rather than what feels good in the moment. This sounds like determination in action. We all know what a disciplined person looks like. How about the Queen's Guards who stand, unflinchingly, in front of Buckingham Palace in London? These guards are disciplined to react only under specific circumstances. Their purpose is to protect the queen. They are true examples of self-control. If they weren't disciplined and instead responded to what felt good in the moment, they'd spend much of their time thwacking annoying tourists. But they know that this isn't right, and their feel-good actions would be frowned upon by the queen.

To have meaning and staying power, discipline needs to come from within us, to ultimately be our choice. Others may teach or guide us, or provide examples, but ultimately discipline is something we decide to do ourselves. The Queen's Guards were taught discipline, but they wouldn't be successful soldiers if their discipline didn't come from within them. Knowing that discipline is our choice gives us more control. Without discipline, we are at the mercy of other people's requests or opinions—more apt to feel like a victim and blame others for our circumstances. As Viktor Frankl says in Man's Search for Meaning, "When we have discipline, we retain control of ourselves and how we move through our environments. When we lose our personal discipline, also our choice, we give control away to other people, external circumstances, and the inevitable randomness of life. Without discipline, we drift and become the plaything of circumstances" (Frankl 2014).

What about discipline and motivation? Is there a similarity? They are related, but they differ. Motivation is the feeling or desire to do something. When we read inspiring stories or quotes about athletes that have accomplished amazing feats, we feel motivated to increase our physical activity. We are excited, and we are ready! We are going to get up tomorrow morning at 5:00 and walk five miles. Then our alarm goes off in the wee hours of the morning, and we look out the window. It is still dark, and it is cold. Our motivation to crawl back under the blankets is now stronger than it is to engage in our physical activity. Motivation is a feeling, and feelings can be inconsistent. Our motivation to walk or move may be high one day and low the next day.

Discipline, on the other hand, is consistent, purposeful practices that align with our purpose. Discipline doesn't depend on our feelings of motivation, though motivation does help. We can delay instant gratification in exchange for greater, long-term rewards. Excuses are the enemy of discipline—and there will always be excuses.

TRAINING OUR BODY IS A METHOD FOR TRAINING OUR MIND

Discipline of our physical body—through movement and healthy nutrition—provides the foundation to further discipline the deeper aspects of ourselves. Let's take the example of getting up at 5:00 am to walk five miles. Now let's say that we have developed discipline to walk at this time regardless of the weather and lack of sunlight. (We should also assume that we have gradually and incrementally worked our way up to such a distance.) We get up to our alarm even though we were in the middle of a wonderful dream. We put on our walking clothes that we'd laid out the previous night. We walk our five miles, we come home and shower, wake our kids, and spend clear-headed time with them while they get ready for school. We are more focused throughout the day because we already got our blood pumping, and we don't have to figure out when we are going to exercise—we've already done it.

We can use the same scenario but assume we did not get up to walk. We awaken to our alarm, annoyed that our dream was cut short. We are still tired, so we snooze the alarm—four more times. Finding us with the blankets pulled over our head, our partner wakes us. We grumpily get up. We begin our day feeling disappointed with ourselves for not following through on our original plan to walk. We shower then wake the kids. We try to multitask by paying attention to the kids and trying to plan a time to walk later in the day. Now we're cranky and distracted throughout the morning; our motivation to walk begins to fade. At lunchtime, we decide we'll just put off our walk until tomorrow. In the afternoon, we choose to eat a piece of chocolate cake that someone brought for their birthday. Perfect timing—we needed an energy boost at that point in the afternoon. Since we were so "off" today, we decide to go for appetizers and drinks with friends before heading home.

Our brains are wired to return to a place of comfort, of stability. If we haven't solidified our disciplines yet or aren't consciously aware of them, it is natural to slip back into our old ways of doing things.

Discipline creates much-needed structure in our chaotic lives. When we discipline our body, we have more control of our mind. Disciplined, routine practices actually free up energy and brain capacity. We don't have to make decisions about these practices; they just become a part of our life. The scenarios we presented weren't advocating doing physical activity only in the morning. They were meant to demonstrate how a lack of discipline in one area of our life can have a domino effect in another area of our life.

Cole had a so-called physical awakening when her kids were young. Her focus and energy were on the children and their needs—a pretty classic mom challenge. She began to feel physically unwell with symptoms of fatigue, low energy, and fuzzy thinking. Though she wasn't sure what was going on, she decided to make one small change. She decided to do some form of daily movement. Once this was solidified into a discipline, she started a daily breath practice. Now she had two disciplines that she was doing for herself. Finally, she started setting her alarm every morning to engage in a morning ritual that involved movement, breathing, and journaling. These disciplines all began and grew incrementally. She discovered she physically and mentally felt better, and her days felt more intentional. And bonus! The benefits of her self-disciplines carried over to her entire family. She became calmer, more patient, more focused, and had more energy to engage with her family in a meaningful way. This is an example of a positive domino effect!

If discipline is a pattern of actions that we routinely follow, think about your daily patterns. Are they intentional? Or are they patterns that you've always followed and never consciously thought about? If we routinely sit on the couch and watch TV from 6:00 until 10:00 every evening, we have subconsciously disciplined ourselves to do that. If we snooze our alarm three times every morning then have to rush to get everyone ready, this is our chosen discipline. We can discipline ourselves to follow patterns that aren't healthy for us, even patterns we'd rather not admit we have. They can be subconscious and unintentional. So, it is important to become aware of our current routines. Let's intentionally choose to keep those that align with our long-term goals.

HOW IS DISCIPLINE REFLECTED IN TRADITIONS?

A number of different traditions teach the importance of discipline, outlining specific behaviors that act as guardrails. Christianity and Judaism have the ten commandments. Buddhism has the five precepts—refrain from taking life, stealing, sexual misconduct, lying, and intoxication. Yoga's Yamas are similar to Buddhist precepts with the addition of non-accumulation. (In modern terms, this means no clutter!) Islam has the Five Pillars of Islam—The profession of faith, daily prayers, almsgiving, fasting during Ramadan, and pilgrimage to Mecca. So, disciplines have played a major part in societies for thousands of years. These guardrails continue to provide boundaries for many of us in our lives. We use them so we don't stray too far off our chosen path.

CHARACTER POWER TOOLS:

Who do we get to become if our mind knows discipline? If we are disciplined, we are more capable of using our power tools. Bonus—our power tools also help us build discipline.

Courage

"Discipline is built by consistently performing small acts of courage" (Sharma 2018). Courage helps us stay the course and persevere through challenges to move along on our path. It takes courage to stand up for ourselves when our friends doggedly beg us to stay out with them until two o'clock in the morning. It takes courage to do what we know is right for us regardless of what people think. We can still value others' opinions yet not submit to them if we are disciplined to do something else.

The opposite of courage may be fear—but it often shows up as complacency and avoidance. When we get complacent and avoid potential discomfort, we eventually become numb. Our lives feel aimless; we feel dependent on others for our own peace and happiness. Our mental and physical health suffer. Mental health symptoms often include procrastination, zoning out in front of the TV or on our devices, overindulgence (overeating, overspending, or being "over-busy"), depression, or anxiety. Physical symptoms may include high blood pressure, stomach aches, headaches, and general lethargy. The lack of courage has its costs. It lowers our quality of life and can affect the lives of our family.

Intellectually, courage can help us analyze our patterns as well as our ingrained beliefs and traditions. After researching and reading about them, what did we learn? Is there anything that we may choose to do differently?

As we've discussed, the lower part of our brain loves instant gratification. Our smartphones, TV, and video games are all readily available and tickling that part of our brain. Discipline requires courage to risk delaying gratification for the sake of a bigger, deeper reward.

Simplicity

The enemies of discipline are distraction, unpredictability, and excuses. If we live chaotic lives, then we are essentially sleeping with the enemies! Start with simple disciplines so the enemies don't have much influence over you. If you want to clean your house, decide on a daily ten-minute cleaning routine. Ten minutes seems doable and sustainable. Rome wasn't built in a day, and it certainly wasn't spotless the next day.

Discipline equals freedom. Routines actually make our lives simpler. They free up our minds, providing more space for creativity and problem-solving. The more straightforward our life is by using simple disciplines, the more liberating our life feels. We have a finite amount of energy—making decisions uses energy. The more we practice our discipline, and it becomes ingrained in our lives, the less energy it takes.

Think of one new discipline that is important to you. Does it relate to a greater goal or purpose? Now how can you strip that down to make it simple and doable? Is it simple enough that it has staying power? Think about how complex we could make a discipline of physical activity. We could introduce our discipline with five hours of high-intensity interval training and weightlifting seven days a week. Simple and doable? How about sustainable? What if we started our physical activity discipline by moving our body for fifteen minutes a day? Is that simple, doable, and sustainable? It most likely is, especially if you are starting a routine.

Positivity

Discipline can naturally have a negative connotation—I have to exercise; or no sugar, no carbs, no pain/no gain. Yet, our brains naturally want to do things that are positive. They want to reject things that are negative. How can we reframe our practice so it is meaningful and positive?

Discipline can seem so serious and regimented. In what ways could we inject humor into our discipline? Let's not be afraid to make routines fun and silly. An example of a simple, light-hearted discipline is the decision to fold laundry with gratitude. Really. Try folding each shirt, sweater, pair of pants, or underwear with love and gratitude—I love you, little t-shirt. You have brought me so much joy. And look at you, little stained pink sweater!

Commitment

Discipline is a commitment with a deep sense of awareness. Commitment is required to get up and show up every day regardless of our motivation. We get up and show up even if we are tired, sick, or injured. Discipline is about being more in tune with our whole body. It is discipline that helps us assess our body and say, "Though we are committed to daily physical activity, we have a pulled hamstring muscle. Today we have to choose swimming over our usual routine of running. Swimming will allow our muscle to heal so we can go on our rock-climbing expedition next month." Discipline helps us connect today's actions with tomorrow's results.

Resilience

We aren't going to be perfect with respect to our practices. We will have times when we want to stop trying. It doesn't help anyone if we beat ourselves up or berate ourselves because we didn't follow through on one of our practices. Remember, discipline is a set of actions that we do on a routine basis. Routinely means regularly, normally, usually, more often than not. Routine is not defined as perfection, rigidity, or inflexibility. When things don't work out, we have an opportunity to assess what happened and learn from the situation. What did we learn? Does this affect the future of our practice, or do we need to tweak something? Did we have a backup plan?

Awareness

When we take a step back and consciously evaluate our current disciplines, we grow our level of awareness. We become aware of the underlying intention that holds that routine in place. Remember, many of the things we are disciplined to are done unconsciously. If we scroll social media for two hours every night, we are very disciplined to that practice. We just may have no idea why. As we bring awareness to our disciplines, we get to choose actions that more closely align to our intentions.

Awareness keeps us focused on our actions and how they relate to our long-term goals. Studies show that distracted shoppers sample more foods at the sampling stations in the grocery store. They also buy more unneeded products from the endcaps of the store aisles. When we are distracted, our brain unknowingly seeks a boost of quick pleasure. Distraction is like a mental roadblock—it blocks our higher-level thinking that connects our present actions with our future goals.

Purpose

Discipline endures for deep-seated reasons, to serve a purpose that we've decided has meaning. It is the force that drives us forward even when our motivation hovers right around zero. Our discipline of reading to the children every night before bed, even when we don't feel like it, has an underlying purpose. Maybe we want our children to associate reading with love and nurturing. Maybe we want them to end their day with a positive, supportive experience. Purpose is one of the key factors that makes discipline persevere.

HOW CAN I PERSONALLY APPLY DISCIPLINE TO MY LIFE RIGHT NOW?

Think about your current daily practices. As you scrutinize each action, ask yourself if that action is steering you in the direction of your choosing. Or is it a distraction, a way to numb out? Are some actions giving you a quick jolt of dopamine to sustain you during your day? Once you've addressed your routines, consider if each one is worth using the finite amount of energy that you have. Is your routine trip to TJ Maxx® helping you with your larger goal of removing clutter from your house—even if that clutter is on sale? Is your discipline of incessantly responding to your smartphone regardless of who you're with helping you with your larger goal of connecting with your family?

How do we become intentional about our disciplines? Where do we start? Can you think of one action that, if made into a routine, would benefit your life? Could your life use daily movement, a morning routine, meal planning, dedicated time with your partner? Once you've made a choice, verify that it is in alignment with your greater purpose.

To be purposefully disciplined, we need to simplify, plan, and focus on what we can control. Instead of starting at square one with something new, what routines are you doing right now that you could merge with your new discipline? Use the power of your current routines to help you maintain your new discipline. For example, if you currently get up at 6:00 am to let the dog outside, incorporate your new discipline of movement to walk your freshly-pottied dog. It is a bonus for both of you! You have an already-established habit of getting up at six in the morning and interacting with your dog. Now you're just adding a step to that routine.

Recall that another way to simplify our lives is to say, "no." If the offer doesn't fit with your set of disciplines or long-term goals, just say no. Consider finding like-minded friends with disciplines similar to yours.

Think about your current environment. Is it conducive to your discipline, or is it distracting? Do you have a treadmill in the basement that you use as a clothesline? If movement is your new discipline, unearth the treadmill and move it to a more inspiring area of your house. Are there distractions or clutter that you can clear in your environment? Are there foods in the house that are tempting? Again, remove temptations and items that are hard to resist.

Plan in advance. We've heard this before—if we fail to plan, we plan to fail. If your new discipline is making healthy weekday meals, lay out a plan for it. On Sunday, plan to look through recipes or online for meal ideas; plan to designate which meals you will have which nights; plan your trip to the grocery store. Then during each evening that week, plan the time you need to start preparing the meal; and plan what part of the meal others can help you with. Without a plan, it is easier to allow our instant-gratification self to take over.

Spend time and energy on things which you can control. You can control your actions, your thoughts, your intentions. Let's go back to our scenario of walking ten miles every morning. The weather is forecasted to be windy and rainy tomorrow morning. We moan to our partner how miserable it will be to walk in such weather. Our mother calls us on the phone from Sunny Acres and asks us how we are doing. We despondently ask her if she's heard about the crappy weather coming our way tomorrow. Seriously, what can we control about the weather? Is there something in ourselves that we can control related to the weather? Maybe our attitude and outlook? We can control what we wear in such inclement weather. We could also control the time we choose to walk. Will it be raining at noon? We don't want to spend precious time and energy trying to control the uncontrollable. And keep in mind, excuses are one of the enemies of discipline.

A fun beat-the-clock type of game you can try is interval training discipline. It involves doing your practice for ten minutes, then taking a five-minute break, then repeat. Take the practice of decluttering. Set your timer for ten minutes. Go all out! Declutter for ten minutes. When the timer beeps, take a 5-minute break. Repeat. Gradually increase the work time if applicable. This exercise can be enjoyable for the whole family as well.

HOW CAN WE USE DISCIPLINE TO STRENGTHEN OUR MARRIAGE?

First of all, be open and honest with each other about any individual routines that are important to you. As partners, how can you be supportive of each other's practices? You might have to get strategic and creative, such as handing off child-care, carpooling, or dinner prep. This is your partner, your best friend, so ask for help if you are struggling with any aspect of your disciplined routine.

Think about the routines that you and your partner currently do together. Are they supporting or strengthening your relationship with each other? Are they supporting the overall goal you two have for your marriage? If you discover that some routines are not adding to the health of your relationship or are stressing it, what could you change? Conscious, positive routines that you do together can be thought of as outward expressions of love. They foster connectedness, growth, and understanding. And what a model you are setting for your children! Remember to add some humor and surprises to your time together. Have some fun.

How about disciplining your thoughts? Can you think of an aspect of your marriage in which disciplining your thoughts may be helpful for your relationship? Do you ever create a story around something your partner does? For example, you come home from a dinner meeting and find the kitchen a mess. Your partner has left the cupboard doors open, the dishes have unidentified food cemented on them, and the dog is licking the inside of the open dishwasher door. An immediate, undisciplined story you may tell yourself is, "My partner is such a slob. They think I can just pick up after them like I have all the time in the world. And look, they forgot to feed the dog, so now the dog is going to get sick from eating leftovers off the dishwasher door!" How much of that story was based on facts? We haven't even talked with our partner yet. The energy it takes to come up with such creative stories in our heads—and we craft them quickly—combined with the resulting emotions can set the tone for the rest of the evening. Can we discipline our thoughts to assume the best in our partner, then ask for clarification of the situation? Consider starting with the phrase, "Help me understand...", then actively listen to their response. This has a deeper, more positive impact on our relationship than simply calling our partner a buffoon.

Partner routines strengthen a marriage because they consist of dedicated time together. Some examples to consider include:

- Two hours of together time every Saturday morning
- Weekly date nights
- Morning yoga or physical activity together twice a week
- Reading in bed together for thirty minutes before going to sleep
- Listening to an audiobook together

HOW CAN WE USE DISCIPLINE TO STRENGTHEN OUR FAMILY RELATIONSHIPS?

Disciplines are actions that express what we value and believe. As we mentioned in the Nutrition chapter, when we have family dinners, we act on our beliefs that shared family time is important. When we read to our children and tuck them into bed at night, we are acting on our belief that interaction with our children includes security, warmth, and affection. Routines are very important to a growing child. In their chaotic little worlds, home routines help them feel safe and grounded.

At the beginning of the chapter, we looked at the many definitions of discipline. A couple of them related to punishment. As we've learned, discipline is the practice of learning, teaching, or training that aligns with a greater purpose. Discipline has a positive focus, one that is based on growth. In regard to using discipline with our children, natural consequences can certainly teach the relationship between our child's chosen action and the resulting effect. But do the consequences provide a teaching moment, an opportunity for growth? Humans, including children, make mistakes. We want to embrace mistakes as a means of learning and growing. We aren't going to cover specific types of discipline because each child is unique, and the range of mistakes kids make requires its own book. We can say that discipline requires patience and energy. It can take some intense thought. But our focus is on long-term success.

Punishment, on the other hand, is meant to cause immediate discomfort as a result of making a mistake. The discomfort is supposed to serve as a memory not to make the same mistake again. Punishment actually requires less thought and energy. We don't have to think about what content we want our child to learn as a result of their mistake. We just raise our voice and send them to their room to "think about what they did." So, what are the possible long-term effects of punishment? Will our child grow up respecting authority without question? Will our child fear authority? Will our child grow up strong and disciplined to follow all rules? What about self-reflection? Does punishment foster critical thinking skills? Does it encourage them to be independent thinkers? Will they be able to say no when their gut or experiences tell them to say no? Finally, is punishment cultivating a long-term, loving relationship with your child?

When we think of purposeful family routines, keep in mind the unique needs of each child. Try to create routines for each child in addition to routines for the whole family. For example, little Margie likes to have her back rubbed every night before bed. Her brother Opie does not like back rubs but prefers to have a goodnight hug before going to sleep. Each child has a different routine, but one that is meaningful to them. Additionally, the whole family participates in practices such as praying before meals as well as brushing teeth and reading before bed.

Other examples of family routines to consider:

- Bedtime routines such as layout clothes for the morning, brush teeth, read stories, good-night kisses.

- Dinner routines such as a gratitude practice: each person talks about three things for which they are thankful

- Family game night once a week

- Dates or one-on-one time with each child: Little Margie gets a date with Mom on Thursday after school. Opie gets his date with Mom on Friday after school.

- Kitchen clean-up after dinners, followed by a family movement activity

- Fun family activity one weekend per month

SUMMARY:

It is easy to think of discipline as something that is challenging or sacrificing of our free will. Discipline is really one of the most freeing and loving things we can do for ourselves. We deliberately choose routines that express our beliefs and will further us on our journey of growth and mastery. We can live more deliberately with more energy and fewer temptations. Having our purpose in mind allows our disciplines to persevere. Remember that discipline takes practice and repetition. Ultimately, the practice will lead to mastery.

CHAPTER 11

MINDSET

The world is falling apart. Boys will be boys. I can't control myself when I eat sweets. I am not creative. Men aren't good at discussing their feelings. Women talk too much about their feelings. People can't be successful unless they graduate from college. My religious belief is the only one that is right and true. These are examples of mindsets. Are these examples facts? Or are they assumptions? It depends on who we ask. Mindsets are deeply held beliefs, attitudes, and assumptions—about who we are and how the world works. It is our routine way of thinking. Our mindset influences the decisions we make, our actions, our health, and how we relate to others.

Our mindset shapes our reality. And no two people share the same mindset.

We may think that we are well-aware of our mindset. We know what we believe. Yet, much of our mindset works below our conscious level. We don't question our subconscious beliefs—we don't even know we have them! Essentially, we are standing firm on unexamined beliefs. So, what are these beliefs and thought patterns? How did they even get created?

Beliefs and mindsets are formed and influenced by our parents, society, and overall environment; and the perceptions we gleaned from personal experiences. Our mindsets officially began forming the moment we were born. As tiny humans, we needed to create a mental model of our world to learn how to survive. At birth, our body contained more than enough brain cells (neurons), but the cells lacked neural connections (synapses) between them. Learning through experience and associations established connections between the brain cells. When we were hungry as an infant, we cried. When we cried, we were eventually fed. As infants, we associated crying with being fed—an early connection between brain cells was made.

The first critical period of brain growth is from age two to age seven. The connections between brain cells double during this time. The brain learns faster than at any other time in our life. So, the experiences that children have during this age range have lasting effects on their memory and development.

Our brain continues to build connections onto existing ones, like branches on a tree. We learn what makes us happy, sad, angry, and scared. We learn who to trust, who to believe. As we learn and grow, our brain looks for patterns to connect new thoughts and experiences to similar ones from our past. Unless we specifically call up our original beliefs and analyze them, they stay submerged. We continue to add branches to our growing tree of knowledge—without observing the quality of our underground roots.

If we don't examine our mindset, we are essentially leading a life scripted by other people. How many of your beliefs are the same as your parents' beliefs? As your teachers' and coaches' beliefs? As your religious institution's beliefs? We carry each of these beliefs until we are brave enough to ask ourselves the question, "Is this belief true for me?" We can also throw in the questions, "Can I think of examples in my life that contradict this belief?" and "Have I used multiple sources to educate myself on this belief?"

Unexamined mindsets can even perpetuate through generations. Are there any negative mindsets we've harbored about particular groups of people? Would they be worth evaluating before we pass them on to our children? Let's look at the complex relationship between Israelis and Palestinians in the Middle East. The two groups have different sets of beliefs and assumptions, and many have witnessed traumatic experiences caused by the opposing sect. The current discord has been going on for generations. Children of Israeli descent have grown up with a mindset that the Palestinians are bad, dangerous people, that the group is the enemy. Children of Palestinian descent have grown up with a similar mindset about the Israelis. Not only does their environment reinforce this mindset, but the children themselves also have witnessed murder and destruction that solidify these beliefs. Could their mindsets ever change?

What do we believe? Where did our beliefs come from? Why do we believe we know some things without a doubt? We'll begin to identify our beliefs, assumptions, and thought patterns— the subconscious rules that we follow. At first, it may feel like we are taking apart a puzzle. Okay, here is an assumption. Why do I believe that? Oh wait, here's another one. Where did that come from? Once they enter our awareness, we can consciously decide if they are constructive, realistic, and in line with where we want to go. If the answer is no, we toss the puzzle piece into the trash. If the answer is yes, then we start putting together a new, more authentic version of our puzzle.

Not surprisingly, even well-examined mindsets have blind spots. How could they not? No two people share the same brain, perspectives, or life experiences. Our mindsets are fragmented ways of looking at the world. They are our own set of filters. Essentially, every person in the world is living their own reality. To appreciate the complexity of ourselves, as well as the different worldviews of others, let's examine how mindsets are created. This can lead to acceptance, understanding, and more peaceful interactions.

A large portion of our mindset was formed by the age of seven. Now consider that the majority of our current daily thoughts are below our conscious level. We are human icebergs! We are only aware of ten percent of our thoughts that hover above the water. Most of those thoughts are the same thoughts we had the day before, and—it is worth noting again—those thoughts are based on a mindset that was developed before we completed second grade! Do you think our mindset is worth examining? Is it time for our own personal intervention?

NEGATIVITY BIAS

We have a genetically wired Negativity Bias. This is a tendency to focus on, learn from, and use negative information far more often than positive information (Vaish et al. 2008, p.383). Let's recall our saber-toothed tiger. If we were out foraging for food and came across a saber-toothed tiger, did we continue looking for food, or did we drop everything and climb the nearest tree? Probably the latter. We tune in to negative information because, historically, it saved our lives! Our brains needed to be on alert, in the red zone, to give our gene pool a chance to survive. Think of the potential outcomes related to our running-saber-toothed-tiger narrative:

If we focused on the negative, "Danger, tiger! Run!", we were more likely to live.

If we ignored our inner negative voice, instead saying, "That is one beautiful tiger! Oh, his stripes are lovely. I wonder if he'd let me pet him.", we were more likely to face an uncomfortable death. And to have our genes plucked from the gene pool.

In our current era in which saber-toothed tigers are extinct, and our food comes from a Frigidaire, how is negativity bias used?

Ask the media.

Negativity bias is used to grab our attention. The media knows how to get people to tune in—and not turn off. Wanting to increase their viewership, they know humans are naturally drawn to negative content, so they provide it. At all hours. Bad things are sudden and exciting. Our brain even releases excitatory chemicals. It further releases a spurt of serotonin if we share the story with others. News sources often repeat similar versions of the same story. So, now we have a negative, repetitive story. How does that affect us? We remember. We create a memory of the story.

When we routinely tune into negative media, our worldview changes. We begin to perseverate on negative content and look for further examples of how bad our world is.

What current negative beliefs do you have about your world right now? Are they facts or opinions nicely dressed as facts? How could your beliefs be wrong?

Let's look at positive news in the media. We don't see a lot of it unless it is sensational: "Woman lifts vehicle off of stranger." Good news occurs more gradually: "The crime rate has decreased in the last year." It doesn't give us that jolt of excitement. It doesn't grab our attention as quickly as negative news. Why? Good, positive news is normal. It happens every day. We just have to turn off the news and look around us. Otherwise, thanks to our negativity bias, negative news will continue to overpower positive "not news."

Jake was once a negativity-bias rock star! About mid-way through Jake's professional hockey career, a coach questioned

Jake about his recurrent bad moods during games. He wondered why Jake would choose a negative mindset over having the mindset of a champion. After some reflection, Jake realized that on game days, he recurrently anticipated negative things to happen. What mistakes might he make? What if his team lost? He thought this mindset was emotionally safer to have than that of a winning mindset. If he thought like a winner and lost the game, he risked being further disappointed than if he just went into the game thinking like a loser.

But our actions follow our mindset. Our brain mentally and physically prepares our body for what we anticipate, what we expect to happen. If we anticipate we are going to fall on the ice, our brain uses its energy to focus on preparing for such a mishap. It continually scans for opportunities to fall. Our brain even releases chemicals and prepares our muscles for a fall. The same process applies when we anticipate something positive. Our brain prepares our body for something good to happen.

For the first time in Jake's life, he understood that mindset could change not only his game of hockey, but also his game of life. Along with the usual rigorous physical training, he began mentally preparing for the results he wanted to see. He visualized, or pictured in his mind, effective plays and team interactions. He even imagined the joyful feelings he would feel when he played well. Jake's physical performance improved—his mindset change allowed him to have the most successful and enjoyable games of his career.

FIXED MINDSET

"We were born with a certain set of natural abilities, traits, and talents. Those will never change. It's a waste of time to spend effort on things I know I'll never be good at doing."

Dr. Carol Dweck, Stanford researcher and author, defined this type of mindset as a "fixed mindset." It describes the little girl who says she doesn't like math class because she isn't good at math. It describes the male college student who delays taking a required art class because "he isn't creative and has never been good at art." Those of us with fixed mindsets create our own limits, ceilings that prohibit us from growing. We attribute our accomplishments to our natural talent and genetic makeup—not hard work and practice.

Typical thought patterns of people with a fixed mindset include:

- There is no point in trying if there is a risk I might fail.
- I stick to what I'm good at.
- I am either good at something, or I'm bad at it.
- Oh, I can't do that. I was never able to....
- When people give me feedback, I feel like they are attacking me. I try to avoid criticism.
- It is what it is. I can't do anything to make this better. I might as well quit.
- I feel resentful or threatened by the success of others. I know I'm not capable of the success others have. They are smarter/better/stronger.

TRUE APPRECIATION OF DIFFERENT MINDSETS

In The Book of Joy, a conversation between the Dalai Lama and Archbishop Desmond Tutu, the two distinguished men discuss eight pillars of joy that cross religion, culture, and time. The first four pillars of joy are qualities of the mind (mindset)—perspective, humility, humor, and acceptance. The book explains that in order to experience joy, we must incorporate these mindsets into our lives.

Perspective begins by stepping back in our minds so we can see the big picture. The Dalai Lama says that for every situation in life, there are many different angles. We must first calm ourselves if we are stressed; our brain can't see perspectives other than our own when we are stressed. We remember that what we think is reality is only part of the picture. When a car cut the Archbishop off in traffic, instead of screaming, "You butthead…and God bless you!", he wondered if the man was rushing to the hospital because his wife was giving birth or someone was dying. Perspective is our choice to reframe our situation more positively. Both men explained that having a wider perspective leads to compassion for others and serenity for ourselves.

Humility is the realization that no one human is better than any other human. The Dalai Lama said,

> [People] should consider me as the same human being, with the same potential for constructive emotions and destructive emotions. When

Let's imagine our friend Sally has a fixed mindset about exercise and her body strength. She thinks that she's always been weak, especially not capable of doing an activity such as weightlifting. We invite her to the gym and together do the assigned group workout—one that involves weights. The workout is hard, and she can't lift as much weight as the majority of others in the class. As we leave, she fights back tears and says, "See! I told you I've always hated exercising, and I just proved that I couldn't lift shit!"

Those of us with fixed mindsets give up more easily and avoid challenges. We know what we're good at doing, and we know what we're "bad" at doing. We create our own box in which to live. Instead of stretching ourselves, we focus our efforts on trying to influence others' opinions of us. "How can I appear smart in this situation? I have to prove to these people that I am good enough to do this project." Do you recognize any of this way of thinking? As we evaluate our own mindsets, it's not uncommon to discover we have a combination of fixed and growth mindsets. We put limits on so many areas of our life when we think we've reached our maximum potential. We sabotage our own health and happiness.

GROWTH MINDSET

Dr. Dweck compared children who displayed fixed mindsets to those with growth mindsets. Children with growth mindsets were more likely to say, "This unit in math is really hard, but we're going to find a way to learn it. We're going to figure it out." People with a growth mindset believe that their mindset is ever-evolving, one that they can continue to develop by learning and practicing.

Those with a growth mindset feel that with enough hard work and practice—regardless of setbacks—they can succeed. In fact, they consider the process as meaningful as the final result. They know that their brain can continue to change and grow when they use it. Challenges are stimulating. Failures are learning opportunities. Perfection does not exist.

Typical thought patterns of people with a growth mindset include:

- I am curious.
- I enjoy the learning process and am excited by challenges.
- I persevere even when I'm frustrated.
- I see effort as a journey, with setbacks a natural part of the path.
- I am inspired by the success of others.
- I like to hang out with and learn from people who are different or smarter than I am.

People with a growth mindset can hold the positive and negative aspects in their minds at the same time. One is not good and the other bad. With endless opportunities, we can develop new skills and continue to improve them throughout our lives. People with a growth mindset focus on the process or the practice, not just the final result. The best musicians, writers, and athletes practice every day. What sets them apart

is their dedication to daily practice—the process rather than the final product. They create micro-goals to master, and they focus on their progress and learning. They live in the present, not wishing away their days until the final product is done.

Cole didn't realize that part of her mindset was fixed until she became familiar with the concept of growth and fixed mindsets. She was always a fan of hard work and effort. She did not embrace criticism or failure—she thought of these as stop signs. Subconsciously her mantra was, "Follow the path of success and approval and thou shalt arrive at the perfect destination." Except she didn't. She found herself following a path to boredom, inauthenticity, and living a story that wasn't hers. She tried to define herself and live according to what she thought she should be—survivor; doctor's wife; devoted mother; immaculate housekeeper; loving sister, daughter, and granddaughter. Even though the story she was living was partially true, she created her script to match how she thought others perceived her. She realized that the story kept her trapped in a mold that was too constricting, keeping her from seeing her own reality. She decided to break out of that mold, to embrace the idea of getting really uncomfortable. To reveal the true person that she was.

Though she still requires some deep breathing to truly appreciate criticism or feedback from others, she now grasps how this information helps her become more—not less.

we meet anyone, first and foremost we must remember that they, too, have the same desire to have a happy day, a happy month, a happy life. And all have the right to achieve it (Gyatso and Tutu 2016, 203).

Humor brings people together. It eases tension and is a sign of trust. The two men do not mean humor that belittles other people. The Archbishop said that humor is about not taking yourself too seriously. Laughing and joking about ourselves "allows us to recognize and laugh about our shared humanity, about our shared vulnerabilities, our shared frailties" (Gyatso and Tutu 2016, 221).

Acceptance is the culmination of perspective, humility, and humor. We acknowledge our current situation. It means seeing a storm and knowing that we have to pass through it. As the Archbishop said, "The acceptance of reality is the only place from which change can begin" (Gyatso and Tutu 2016, 224). We accept that we will have periods in our lives that will be difficult as well as periods that will be peaceful, and we will respond in the best way we can. A positive growth mindset gave the Dalai Lama and Archbishop Desmond Tutu hope and a greater perspective to make the world a better place.

Let's return to the situation about the Middle East. Networks do exist with a focus on peace that consist of both Palestinians and Israelis. One such partnership is called "Friends of Roots." Its goal is to develop an understanding of each other despite their differences, to appreciate different perspectives and mindsets. They mutually recognize and respect each People's connection to the Land. The partnership gives the local people an opportunity to have some control, some responsibility—to change their society (www.friendsofroots.net). Their work is aimed at challenging the assumptions their communities hold about each other, mindsets that have been generational. These courageous people decided to examine and question their mindsets. They chose not to perpetuate their ancestors' beliefs without personally examining them for themselves!

MINDSET REFRAMING

Our mindset shapes our experiences and our reality. Mindset reframing begins when we explore our deeply held beliefs, assumptions, and thought patterns. We decide whether or not to keep them. We then begin the process of creating new thought patterns that will be helpful to us—ones that will help us grow personally and within our relationships. The latter will take dedicated practice, though, as our patterns in our relationships are pretty well-established. But we can do it. We will be uncomfortable for a bit, but we know this feeling will fade. We will survive. If we change our mindset, we change our lives! Grab a pen and journal.

Breath Practice

The breath acts like a bridge that connects our body, mind, and spirit. Breath practice regulates the body in such a way that it also quickly calms the mind. It helps us separate ourselves from our thoughts. We are then able to witness these thoughts, ultimately noticing our patterns of thinking.

Using the breath is a very effective way to get to a meditative state. It is used in a number of practices. Meditation is one such practice that has been well-researched. Studies have shown that meditation actually changes the structure of our brains. Researchers found more connections between brain regions in people who meditated. They also found reduced activity in the "me" center (the prefrontal cortex) of the brain. Being present in a meditative state allows us to see things more clearly, creates a sense of calm, enhances compassion, and puts the brakes on pain and anxiety.

Breath practice and meditation can help us assess how our mindsets play out in our lives. From there, we can begin to question those patterns and their underlying beliefs and assumptions. What do they mean? How do I currently act on them? Where did I learn them? Are they helpful or positive? Are they limiting? Is my family benefitting from them? Finally, we can ask ourselves, "Do I want to continue this thought pattern?"

Growth Mindset

Life is a series of adventures and misadventures. Let's embrace them and learn as we go. Practice growth-mindset thinking. Rehearse it during your meditation, on your walk, or on your drive to work. Once you've repeated it multiple times on your own, use it in an area of your life that is uncomfortable.

1. Identify your beliefs and assumptions.

   Schedule some time alone on a regular basis to focus on your breath. Do not judge yourself during these practices. You may want to bring up beliefs or assumptions by subject, for example:

   - What are my beliefs about my weaknesses?

   - What are my beliefs about failure, about success?

   - What are my beliefs about breath practice and mindfulness?

   - What are my beliefs about prayer and religion? How about other faith practices?

   When a belief or assumption arises, name it. Write it in your journal.

2. Evaluate your beliefs and decide whether or not to keep them.

   Once you have some written down, look at the beliefs one at a time. Ask yourself the following questions:

   - Is this belief negative or positive (or neutral)?

   - Does this belief add value to my life and relationships?

   - Is this an example of a fixed mindset or a growth mindset?

   - Is this belief based on fact or opinion?

- How could I be wrong about this belief?

3. Practice new patterns of thinking.

   - Acknowledge we have choices in how we think. As we get more adept at recognizing our thoughts, we can consciously choose the direction we'd like to go.

   - Replace the word "failing" with "learning."

   - Add the word "yet" to something that you don't know how to do.

   - Get out there and try new things, not just those things you already know that you like. Don't limit yourself. Consider stretching yourself. Risk doing something uncomfortable.

   - Reflect on how much you've learned or grown in previous endeavors—driving a car, raising children, cooking. We didn't just quit when we made a mistake.

   - Stay authentic. Be vulnerable. Stop looking for approval. We give up our opportunities to learn and grow when we focus on the approval of others.

   - Reframe criticism as "helpful instruction." It is a free learning opportunity. We always have room to improve. "Room to improve" does not mean failure.

Positivity

Since our brains are naturally wired to see potential danger or negativity, we need to put some real effort into seeing the positive. We can re-wire our brains to embrace the positive, but it will take determination and daily practice. But the practice can be oh-so-worth-it! It is like a veil being lifted from our eyes—we will see the good and the beauty without our negativity filter.

When we talk about positivity, we aren't advocating a Polly-Anna-like mentality. We still observe the real world; we just want to alter our focus. Our brain naturally looks for patterns to associate with our past experiences. We want to balance our tendency to look for negative patterns with a new practice of looking for positive patterns. And what does that bring us? Like a simple math equation, adding a positive to a negative equals a neutral, right? Not in this case. Research has shown that it takes five positive thoughts to neutralize one negative thought. Five-to-one is the magic ratio we need to overcome our negativity bias! We can apply this ratio of thoughts and interactions to our marriage and family relationships as well. Five positive interactions with our partner or child will begin to disintegrate the one sticky, negative interaction. We then arrive at neutral, which is where we want to be. We can pat ourselves on the back for doing some heavy lifting in the positivity arena!

Gratitude practice

When we practice gratitude, we notice the little gifts in life—not just the monumental ones, but those that are so often overlooked. When such gifts are woven together, they create a netting that catches positive thoughts. We need to hoard our positive thoughts. As neuroscientist Rick Hanson wrote, "Most positive experiences flow through the brain like water through a sieve, while negative ones are caught every time" (Hanson 2013). Negative thoughts are just stickier than positive thoughts.

How can we practice gratitude and accumulate our positive thoughts?

- Find something to be grateful for when you first wake up in the morning and right before you sleep at night. To make them even stickier, write them in your journal.

- "Bookmark" positive experiences in your mind. Specifically, remember details of the positive experience and rehearse them in your mind. This helps create a memory that sticks.

- Search for the silver lining—actually, five swatches of it—in negative or mundane situations. This doesn't mean you ignore your uncomfortable feelings in difficult situations, nor does it mean living in a state of denial. You just don't want the negative feelings to control you. Think of five positive effects that might result from one negative situation. Even if the positive thoughts are bizarre or silly, we are training our brain to look for the good, for the opportunities, for ways to grow.

Gratitude practice goes beyond mindset training. It teaches us that we can be content even when things aren't overtly "going our way." It improves our mental health and our relationships.

Physical activity

Physical activity can help rewire our mindset toward positivity. As we've discussed, physical activity creates chemical changes in our brains and releases feel-good endorphins. Not only does this chemical release promote positivity, but it also helps us think more clearly, learn more easily, and make better decisions—all very useful in reframing our mindsets.

To capitalize on our exercise endorphins, we can add fun and humor to our physical activities. Laughter also releases positive brain chemicals. Bonus!

Stretching releases endorphins as well. We can all make time to stretch throughout the day. As Cole learned in yoga, "Through the body, we can put a brake on the mind." When Cole restarted her movement activities, her mental fog dissipated. Other benefits soon followed: increased motivation, positivity, and energy.

Physical activity helps shift the energy of negative thoughts, allowing us to recognize the positives in life.

HOW IS MINDSET REFLECTED IN TRADITIONS?

Mindset has been emphasized in a number of different religions and traditions. They all highlight the importance of examining our thoughts. While some religions are unyielding in how we form our mindset and what the result should be, other religions and traditions focus on a mindset of peace, calm, and acceptance.

The Yoga Sutras describe yoga as calming the endless motion of consciousness. It refers to creating a still mind, taming the pinball-like patterns of thoughts in our head. Mind training is a foundational aspect of Buddhism. Buddha stated, "The mind is everything. What you think, you become." He also stated in the Dhammapada, "With our mind, we create our own world."

Christianity refers to training our mind on God or the Holy Spirit. In broad terms, this is training our mind to get out of our heads—to focus on a higher power whose essence is positivity (love, joy, peace, self-control, kindness, mercy, grace).

Judaism exemplifies a growth mindset through confessional during Yom Kippur. Though they enumerate their misdeeds, they do so knowing that God forgives their mistakes if they learn from them. Growing from their mistakes allows them to be better tomorrow than they were yesterday.

Islam views thinking as an act of worship. Sustaining a healthy mind and an effective state of thinking is integral to the faith.

CHARACTER POWER TOOLS

A positive growth mindset can strengthen our character power tools. We realize that we can change and continually evolve our character. Our character is not set in stone. Each of our power tools can, in turn, help us examine our current beliefs and mindset. They can further help us reframe it and develop it into a growth mindset.

Courage

A growth mindset is essentially a practice of courage. We take on challenges that may involve numerous attempts before we ultimately succeed. Think about performing a pull-up for the first time. We had an initial belief that we could never do a pull-up. However, with our new growth mindset, we've decided not to limit ourself in such a way. So, we start out slowly, using three stretch bands around a pull-up bar. We perform ten banded pull-ups once a week. As we get stronger, we remove one of the stretch bands and increase our reps. Since we celebrate micro-goals, we celebrate when can do a pull-up after removing one of the stretch bands. How many tries does it take before we thrust our chin above the bar without a stretch band? It can take more than a year of practicing pull-ups before achieving the first unassisted pull-up. But, wow, we accomplished something we always told ourselves that we could never do!

Mindset reframing requires courage—courage to focus on something new and courage to consistently practice. Jake equated his daily, rigorous, physical training to the training of his new mindset. Both involve deliberate focus and hard practice. But when game time arrives, our trained mindset springs into action.

Negative patterns and fears have established pathways in our brain. This is why they come naturally to us, even if they aren't helpful. Gossiping is an example of a normalized, negative activity. It takes courage to decide to leave an easy and comfortable pattern, such as gossiping with our friends. Choosing a new mindset will not be comfortable at first. "Gossiping is what we've always done when we get together. What will we talk about? This could be really uncomfortable." That is okay. We really can survive being uncomfortable for a bit. The feeling will dissipate as we form our new pattern.

Simplicity

Our minds have a natural tendency to make things more complex. Remember how we like to add narration to situations? We need to consider the whole situation, then break it down into what are facts and what is narrative. Next, we decide which facts we can control. Related to mindset reframing, we begin by using small, simple steps—daily tasks and micro-goals. Consider picking one thought to work on at a time.

Examining our mindset and consciously choosing our beliefs declutter our mind. We can drastically reduce the mental clutter that stunts our growth:

- How can I be all things to all people?
- What will people think?
- I wish someone would tell me what I'm supposed to do next!

Reducing such clutter will give our brain more bandwidth to focus on what we know is important. At the present time.

Positivity

Training the brain to reframe our thoughts and inputs requires us to be on the lookout for positivity. Though our media magnifies conflict twenty-four hours a day, we can look around and easily see examples of social harmony. A nice family dinner. A sports team that supports each other. A healthy relationship with a friend or coworker. A stranger who picks up someone else's trash. Positivity helps us become solution-oriented rather than crisis-focused.

As we learned, our mind needs five times more positive input than negative input just to arrive at neutral thinking. The media make a profit from negative stories. How can we seek the positive to offset this negativity? We can schedule time each day to tune in and turn off the media. We can also look for "good news" media sites. And we know that creating a daily routine of conscious gratitude is a simple, no-cost way to practice positivity.

A positive mindset can change a potentially contentious situation into one of contentment. We can practice positive thinking before an anxiety-provoking event or situation—rehearse a positive outcome in our mind then visualize it.

Commitment

We each have an incomplete and biased mindset. We continue to take in new information and experiences then connect the dots to the known information inside our heads. It takes commitment to deconstruct and unlearn some of our long-term beliefs. Because they have been pervasive in our lives, our beliefs can show up in many areas. Commitment to the process recognizes that we can't change these beliefs overnight. It will require ongoing work, not a one-time quick fix.

We adults are not starting from a blank slate like children do when they begin to make neural connections. Our connections are so well-used and so efficient that avoiding them feels like a threat to our survival. (Graziano Breuning 2016, 118) This is why change is hard for adults. But we can learn and create new connections by persistent repetition.

Resilience

Training our thoughts to find the good in situations is a practice in resilience. Resilience is buoyed by hope—knowing that, even in dark times, there will be good in the future. Training our mind on positivity and letting go of our old thought patterns strengthens our ability to persist in other areas of our lives as well.

Being resilient requires flexibility in old thinking patterns. We don't need to think of problems as dead-ends. We can think of them as bumps in the road, as challenges, as ways to grow. We have an opportunity to look for other ways to solve problems. Life isn't black or white. We don't have to think of mistakes as only failures. Right or wrong thinking is limiting. We need to give ourselves some grace and a high-five for learning. Flexible thinking provides us with freedom and space to try and try again.

Awareness

Increasing awareness allows us to see a thought as just that—a thought. It is not our identity. For example, we observe our thought, I am so awkward around large groups of people as simply a thought. We can choose to keep that thought or leave it behind. We can also acknowledge our thought patterns, challenge them if necessary, then disrupt the patterns that are consistent with a fixed or negative mindset. As we progress in our awareness, we can even observe when we slip into a fixed or negative mindset, then correct ourselves mid-course.

Awareness is required to recognize when we are in a negative spiral, one in which we keep repeating the negatives so often that we forget a positive is even possible.

It's often easier to diagnose someone else's mindset, even try to change them. This is a great opportunity for conflict! Let's remember that we add our own narrative to others' unique mindsets. And we can't exactly know someone else's mindset—we can't enter their brain. We can, however, question our narrative. What is factual, and what is an assumption?

Purpose

If our purpose is to remain exactly the same in a world we cannot change, then all we need is a fixed mindset. We wouldn't even want to read this book! If we believe we can continue to learn more, love more, and become more, we're on the growth mindset path. Consider how a change in mindset might affect our marriage, our children, our grandchildren? If purpose is the driving force behind the meaningful work we do for ourself and others, does our current mindset equip us for that work? Or does our mindset need a little rewiring?

HOW CAN I APPLY MINDSET TO MY PERSONAL LIFE?

We need to remember that we are not locked into the belief system in which we grew up. We can change!

- Start by thinking about one fixed belief that you have about yourself. Complete the statement, "I just can't...." Now work on changing that one belief and turning it into a growth mindset. An example of a fixed mindset is "I just can't learn a new language. I've never been good at learning languages." If we turn it into a growth mindset, it may look like, "I know I can learn a new language. I'm very interested in learning German. I may need to try different methods of learning, but I will commit to practicing it every day."

- When you feel fearful or anxious, remember the phrase, "I am not a caveman, and this is not a tiger."

- When positive events happen, repeat them in your mind. We tend to let positive events flow right through us, and we allow negative thoughts to stick to us like Velcro.

- Keep a journal. Write down three to five things that you are thankful for each day.

- Create and accept opportunities that push you out of your comfort zone. This pushes you toward a growth mindset.

HOW CAN WE USE MINDSET TO HELP STRENGTHEN OUR MARRIAGE?

- Think about the mindsets that surround your marriage. What beliefs and assumptions did you each bring into the marriage? Think about the issue of conflict. Do you think of conflict as a warning sign that your marriage may be in trouble? Or do you look at conflict as an opportunity to make positive change?

- Think about flexibility. Are you in a marriage that has a rigid set of rules? Or is your marriage more adaptable? Think about the need for approval or validation from your partner. These are fixed mindset qualities. To change them to growth mindset qualities, we need to find validation within ourselves.

- Practice gratitude with your partner. Explicitly tell your partner what it is about them for which you are thankful. Knowing that it can take five positive thoughts to neutralize one negative thought, some of us need to start identifying the positives. Like anything else, the more we practice gratitude and the more we look for the positives, the easier this will be.

- Praise your partner's efforts. We know that we should praise a child's efforts, not their abilities. Do we do that in our marriage?

- What if you and your partner both have a growth mindset but don't share the same mindset? Can you address differences with curiosity and questions rather than judgment? "How interesting! Tell me more about what you mean by that." This shows respect for the other person's beliefs by wanting to find out more about them. Just think, your children are more apt to grow up knowing it's okay to ask questions. Addressing differences in mindsets is an opportunity to practice conflict in constructive ways.

HOW CAN WE USE MINDSET TO STRENGTHEN OUR FAMILY RELATIONSHIP?

As parents, when we praise our children's efforts rather than abilities, we put a positive emphasis on learning. As Dr. Dweck says, "If parents want to give their children a gift, the best thing they can do is to teach their children to love challenges, be intrigued by mistakes, enjoy effort, and keep on learning. That way, their children don't have to be slaves of praise. They will have a lifelong way to build and repair their own confidence" (Dweck 2016).

How to nurture a growth mindset in our children:

- Remind your children that making mistakes is a normal part of life. Everybody on this planet makes mistakes!

- Emphasize practice, effort, and progress rather than the final result.

- If your child says something with absolute certainty, yet it's an obvious opinion, you can help them become aware of their own thoughts. Consider saying, "That's interesting. What makes you think that? Do you think that is always the case?"

- Identify some of your mistakes in front of your children. Role model positive self-talk after your mistake.

- Use an activity to show mistakes as growth. Give everyone a piece of paper. Ask them to write (or draw) something that they think they've failed at. Have them crumple up the paper like they are getting rid of the failure. Now have them open the paper and write down what they learned from the "failure." Ask them if they think it was a failure since they learned from it. This is an opportunity to reinforce replacing the word "failure" with "learning." When we make mistakes, we grow our brains.

- Consider giving each child their own gratitude journal. At bedtime, you can encourage them to think about their day. What are they thankful for? Your child can either draw or write what they are thankful for in their journal.

- Another gratitude practice can occur during family meals. As you go around the table, ask each person to name something that happened that day for which they are thankful.

- Provide an example that shows how positive thoughts can overpower negative thoughts. Place a drop of water-color paint (negative thought) in a bowl of water (positive thought). Show your children that the color is very strong at first. Have them continue to watch the color. Eventually, it mixes in with the water, and you can't see it anymore.

SUMMARY

Our mindset guides our pattern of thinking and actions. It influences how we see the world and how we influence others. We established our mindset at a young age—a result of our experiences, and the beliefs and opinions of those influential people in our lives. To continue to refine ourselves on our journey, we need to be open to unlearning ideas and beliefs that no longer serve us.

When we try something new or challenging, we risk failing. We also risk sprouting new wings and flying! It takes courage to say, "I can keep trying. I am capable of finding another way."

Regardless of the set of beliefs we grew up with, we can now determine if we want to claim these beliefs as our own. It is not too late to learn, and it's not too late to change. We have not reached our limits. A growth mindset says that we are good, and we can be better. Challenges, practice, and repetition— bring it on!

SECTION IV

THE SPIRITUAL SELF

Spirituality is a connection to something greater than ourself. It is personal—it consists of a different path for everyone. Religion, God, a higher power or force, nature, a sense of connectedness are all examples of spirituality. It is an awareness that increases feelings of hope, trust, and perseverance. Now that we know how to care for our physical bodies and focus our minds, we can overlap these more tangible components with our spiritual awareness. Spiritual awareness can creep into every crevasse of our physical and psychological body. Spirituality is looking inside ourself to notice a great source of strength and connection.

Spiritual connections foster potential health benefits. They boost the feel-good, mood-stabilizing serotonin levels in the brain. They increase motivation. Studies have also shown that spiritual beliefs or rituals help heal our physical body.

Spirituality is not rigid. It is not about dogma. It is beautiful and nonjudgmental. There are many paths of spirituality to explore. It is a feeling like a greater power has our back as we journey through this life.

CHAPTER 12

CONNECTION

Connection spans so many entities—from connecting to all aspects of our Self, to the Divine, and to other people. It also includes the interconnected nature of things in the world, the interdependence among all of us. What really is connection as it relates to building and strengthening our Self?

Is connection a relationship of cause and effect? "Running six miles made my legs feel wobbly and my mind feel clear." or "Sitting on the couch eating licorice while binge-watching Netflix all day made me feel sluggish and slightly nauseated." We're already experiencing the connection our physical body has with the rest of our Self. Movement and nutrition have a causal relationship with our physical and mental health.

Is connection an awareness of something within ourselves, such as our inner voice or relationship with the Divine? "During our interview with George for a new staff position, I continually felt a nagging sensation that George was hiding something. It was a gut feeling." or "When I hiked to the top of the Continental Divide, I looked all around me and experienced a profound sense of connection to our earth and to the Divine." This deep awareness is a connection to our internal guidance, to something that feels greater than ourselves.

Is connection an intimate relationship with another person or group? "I feel deeply connected to my family and close friends. I trust them enough to tell them anything; I can be vulnerable with them." Humans are born with the need for connection. Each one of us needs to feel like we belong— somewhere and to someone.

Is connection recognition that we are all linked as human beings? The group of Israeli and Palestinians in the Friends of Roots realized that they were all humans who experienced similar emotions such as joy, sadness, and fear. Both groups wanted safety and a better future for their children. They bonded over shared emotions and a sense of compassion.

In our era, the COVID-19 pandemic helped us realize the importance of connection and community, at all levels. We were forced to recognize our mortality and the effects of death and loss. We lost precious connections, parts of ourselves. And due to the causal relationship between exposure to and contracting the disease, many who were sick had to suffer alone. Yet, this was an unanticipated opportunity to change the way we connected with people. We deepened our connections with some people and let other, more shallow relationships go. We felt new connections to people we didn't even know—people with whom we had never exchanged words—but shared in our struggles and frustrations. We connected with others as we took on new roles: as caregivers, teachers, and counselors; or simply as a person struggling, grieving, or lost. We realized that amid struggle, connecting with others helped us heal. It was like salve on a wound. Physiologically, a feeling of connection slows the release of the stress hormone cortisol, in our brain. The result is a much-needed sense of calm. And this was necessary during such a time of uncertainty.

To truly have deep, genuine connections with others, it is important to have a connection with ourselves first. This is called our authentic or true self, our intuition, our inner voice. We have discussed the process of getting in touch with our inner voice as it relates to our physical self and our mind. Our spiritual connection weaves its way among the previous two, like a web. When we discover and trust our authentic self, we can be open to a healthy connection to a higher power, to our loved ones, and to humanity in general.

CONNECTION TO OURSELVES

We essentially have two inner voices that are very different from each other, oftentimes at odds with each other: our ego and our intuition. We need both of them, but we need them to work together harmoniously. Our ego is our thoughts, our logical mind, and it is heavily influenced by the world around us. It serves to give us an individual human experience, but it is a drama queen! It often operates out of fear and scarcity. It likes to control situations. It loves to blame others and feels fulfilled through sources outside ourselves—shopping, alcohol, and other people. The ego is our conscious should and shouldn't voice. We should look both ways before we cross the street. We shouldn't dive off a cliff until we know how deep the water is. Most significantly, the ego seeks comfort and pleasure, and it perseverates on what others think of us.

Our intuition—our authentic self, our inner voice, our soul, Chi—is our awareness behind the scenes. It is our gut feeling. It comes from the heart. We just know something without having a logical reason or explanation. Intuition is our connection to the Divine. It is love and acceptance of ourselves. It is not judgmental and doesn't look to outside sources for fulfillment or validation. Our intuition is decisive. It helps us know exactly what we need. It doesn't need to control a situation or others' opinions of us.

Unfortunately, we've been conditioned to keep our intuition quiet.

Our society values and acts on the logical mind. We need facts. We need proof. We need solid evidence. Learning to connect with our intuitive mind, this deeper, whole part of ourselves, helps us let go of our egoic structures and express ourselves from a place of love and truth.

Both our ego and intuition are important, but we need a balance. As humans, we have the benefit of running our intuition through our logical mind. For example, our intuition tells us to run across the street to comfort a child who just fell off their bike. Our logical, egoic self remembers we should look for traffic before running across the street. A symbiotic relationship can exist.

Since our ego tries to defend us from hurt and pain, it stays busy scanning for possible threats. "I think those people are gossiping about me! Do they know I've just been fired from my job? Should I say something or just appear angry and aloof?" Listening to our ego-based thoughts can be utterly exhausting—but only when we feed them, when we continue to believe them without question. When we get to know our authentic self, we realize that we are not our thoughts. Our thoughts do not define us. We are the vastness beneath our thoughts. We are like the depth of the ocean, our thoughts like the waves on its surface. Our authentic self has no fear and does not try to impress anyone. It is love. It is truth. It is whole. And we each have it within us. We simply have to connect to it and listen to it.

Unfortunately, our ego thinks it the star of the show.

It's time for our authentic self and ego to have a little chat. How can they work together? The best way to hear our intuition is by making space through mindfulness or breath practice. Keep in mind, our ego is loud and will try to overpower our intuitive inner voice. We can reassure our ego that we still need it, but it can now be the follower. With our authentic self moving into the lead, it can now nudge, question, and guide our egoic thoughts. As we become aware of our authentic self, we can begin operating from that level. We can decipher whether our thoughts are coming from our ego or intuition. Our ego might say, "I need to be recognized and praised for what I've done!" or "I need to prove to my coworkers that I can do this project." Our authentic self helps us become aware of those thoughts and agree with them or contradict them. Our ego and authentic self are like a system of checks and balances. They are both needed, but both need to be examined and clarified.

Jake talks about how his connection with his authentic self didn't happen right away. It did not come at age twenty when he was partying and hungry for power on the ice. Far from it. At that time in his life, he said he wouldn't have chosen to be friends with himself, let alone listen to his inner voice. He constantly lived in a heightened state of anxiety, preoccupied and worried about proving himself to other people. This is why he felt mentally spent by the end of each day. So, in the evenings? Hello, beer—what a delightful distraction and numbing agent! That only lasted so long. After professional hockey became a memory, Jake realized he needed something deeper, something purposeful. Tools from retired Navy Seal Commander Mark Divine as well as the discovery and growth in his faith helped him discover his authentic self. Today, he practices connecting to his true self and his purpose every morning. He prays. He makes a deep dive to assess what his inner voice is saying. Is the voice positive and action-oriented? He listens. Are negativity and fear trying to creep in? He dives deeper. Jake says that historically, the last person he was accountable to was himself. He couldn't figure out why he felt so emotionally crushed when he let others down. Yet, he let himself down all the time. His cup was empty, and he relied on others to fill it.

He still appreciates what was once his numbing agent of choice, Budweiser®, but it is no longer his crutch. It is no longer needed as a way of shutting off his internal chaos.

Without a connection to a deep understanding of ourselves, how can we create such a connection with others? Our ego doesn't really know what we want, though it thinks it does. If we made a connection with someone else before knowing our authentic self, the relationship may be between our ego and the other person. Our connection would be based on who best could fulfill our emotional needs, who could fill our cup. This is not an indication of an enduring relationship between two people. By developing a patient, loving relationship with ourself first, we are able to give love to others. It is one of the most generous gifts we can bring to a relationship with another person.

CONNECTION TO A HIGHER POWER

A relationship with the Divine is a connection to something greater than ourself. It is personal and consists of a different path for everyone. This is different than organized religion. God, Breath, a higher power, Source, Allah, Yahweh, the Universe, and Mother Earth are all examples of sources of spiritual connectedness. This relationship increases feelings of hope, trust, and perseverance. We are able to sit with fear and uncertainty while knowing our source of strength comes through and from within us.

Our brains are positively affected by a connection to a higher power. Research from the journal Social Neuroscience shows that religious and spiritual experiences can activate the brain's reward circuits in the same way as love, sex, gambling, drugs, and music (Ferguson et al. 2018). In fact, an entire field of study is dedicated to the interaction of religion and our brain—Neurotheology.

What is this power bigger than us, the Divine? It is hard to concretely define because it is on a spiritual plane. Our personal higher power may not make sense to other people. That's okay. It is personal—our ego is the only one concerned with what other people think anyway. Our higher power is our guidance. We are deferential to something bigger than ourselves. Instead of aiming to control everything ourselves, we ask for support from the Divine. This spirit leads us toward a more present, patient, loving, grounded, and joyful way of being.

Connection to our authentic self enables us to become aware of a higher power. To listen. To decipher. Our true self also protects us from becoming intimidated or hurt by the dogma attributed to some religions. Author Glennon Doyle says that God or higher power means breath. "We are always close to our breath. If we feel lost, we know how to return to our breath. Many institutions don't want us to know that in order to connect to God, we just have to breathe" (Doyle 2020, 240). We are connected to our higher power through our heart and mind. If a religious leader says that they speak for God and that without question, we should believe their words—isn't that telling us to mistrust our own connection with the Divine?

Jake and Cole are both very spiritual and have fulfilling connections with God. However, their higher powers look different. Jake's higher power is Jesus Christ. Jake connects with Jesus via prayer, and he connects with Jesus' teachings by reading the Bible. He does this every morning after taking time to breathe and meditate to connect with his authentic self. A hierarchy of connections works best for Jake. He checks in with himself first to assess his mindset. This prepares him for his connections: Me with my Faith, Me with my Wife, Me with my Kids. He says that if any of those connections get out of whack, the results just cascade down through the links.

Cole is a practicing Catholic, though her lens on faith also includes eastern traditions. Her strongest connection is with the Holy Spirit, the aspect of the Divine that lives within us. Through this connection, she unites with her authentic self. Her connections to her authentic self and spirit are just as critical to her as connections with others. Each morning through meditation and breathing, she connects to what is happening in her body and mind. She has strengthened her connection with the Holy Spirit through meditation, breathing, prayer, and visualization. These are the grounding forces that allow her to make meaningful connections with others throughout the day.

CONNECTION WITH OUR LOVED ONES

What do you think of when you hear, "We have a wonderful relationship, a solid connection"?

Deep, but simple exchanges?

Healthy interdependency?

Non-judgmental presence?

Safety?

Soulmate?

Shared values?

Ability to finish each other's sentences?

Think of connections between people as bonds, the toothpicks we once used to link gum-drop molecules during our fourth-grade science experiment. Two green gumdrops of hydrogen connected with one purple gumdrop of oxygen. Unique elements, but when connected, they form another unique element—water. When two humans, who each have strengths of their own, make a connection, the result is a whole new creation. The possibilities! A melding of ideas, using each other's individual strengths to uncover deeper meanings, to discover solutions, to better understand ourselves and the world.

Scientists continue to investigate the health benefits of connecting with other people. They've found that connection reduces both stress and the hormones that cause stress. This affects our immune system, insulin regulation, gut function, and arteries that lead to our heart. Social connection also keeps our memory sharp, especially in older people. Studies show that senior citizens who are socially connected are happier, have more physical mobility, and have a lower risk of dementia. The centenarian Blue Zone research suggests that connection makes up one-third of the factors related to living a long life (Buettner 2012). A connection with family, friends that support healthy practices, and a faith-based community are factors that lead to a longer life. Just think, we can become the older, wiser members of society someday—the ones who can still play on the floor with their great-great-grandchildren!

On a very different note, chronic loneliness can make us more prone to illnesses and ultimately have a shorter lifespan. People who are not socially connected are more likely to smoke, be inactive, have high blood pressure, and be overweight. Their hope, happiness, and quality of life are less than they could be with a sense of belonging. Many think the answer to loneliness is social media. Unfortunately, rather than feeling more connected to others via social media, people feel disconnected and lonelier. Social media exhibits people smiling, having fun, being silly, and celebrating together. Our ego sees this and screams, "Why isn't my life like that?"

We are wired for connection, even those of us who swear to be profound introverts. Our core biological and psychological need for connection begins at birth—through a relationship with our caregiver. Children who have connections during their early years are more likely to have healthy relationships when they grow up. The Grant Study, a Harvard research project that followed nearly 300 men for over seventy years, found that the best predictors of physical health, economic success, and a happy life were intimate connections—loving childhoods, capacity for empathy, and warm relationships as young adults.

"Connections are relationships that go beyond the surface and help us feel heard, understood, supported, and even celebrated" (Battle 2017). We can almost feel the words from this quote. Meaningful interactions bring us joy and contentment. The quality of relationships matters.

Cole describes her early adult life as one that was easy to balance, being an independent introvert who enjoys deep, meaningful connections. Until she arrived at motherhood. Complete sensory overload. Sleep-deprived, she started her day when the first child stirred, and she continued her day in a reactive mode, like zone defense, letting the children's needs dictate her day. She felt she was just drifting through her days, being carried along with the current of busyness. She realized she had been overlooking the most important connection—the connection to herself. She worked hard to cultivate time alone so that when she was with her family, she was able to operate on a full battery. She could then nourish the connections that mattered most to her.

The most intimate connections we have are with our partner and our children. Remember the za-za-zing that we felt when our relationships were new—a new love in our life, a new baby? The initial buzz eventually fades to a slow hum in all relationships. When this occurs, those that solely rely on others for their contentment begin to feel restless. They need something or someone else to feel fulfilled again. This may include a new partner, an affair, or another baby. How can we stop this type of cycle? How can we freely give and receive love when we are already in a valuable, steady relationship? The feeling of fulfillment needs to come from within us. Failure to connect with ourself leads to failure of long-term connections with others. If we aren't acquainted with our authentic self, who is making the connection with the other person? Our ego? Healthy relationships begin with us knowing our authentic self. Deeper relationships with others will follow— relationships that are true and lasting.

How do we connect and show our love to our loved ones? Do we demonstrate it in the same way to all of them? Family members may have different ways they'd like to experience connection. One of our children wants to be physically cuddled, hugged, and kissed before bed every night. The more physical contact, the better. Our other child prefers quality time reading with us. Our partner lights up when we acknowledge how much we love them and appreciate what they do for our family. A book written in the 1990's yet is still relevant today discusses five general preferences of giving and receiving love. The book is called The Five Love Languages by Gary Chapman. The Love Languages Gary describes are Words of Affirmation, Acts of Service, Receiving Gifts, Quality Time, and Physical Touch. When you think about yourself, is there one general category that you gravitate to? If so, have you let your partner know this? If you still aren't sure, an online quiz is available if you'd like to dig deeper. The quiz is available at www.5lovelanguages.com. This concept of love languages provides a general idea of how we can connect best with each family member.

Connection weaves humans together, although we each keep our individual identity. A healthy connection sends the message that we value the relationship even if we don't agree with or understand the other's thoughts or actions. The relationship is deeper than the subject matter. Practicing this is not easy, especially for parents. When our adolescent daughter surprises us by dying her hair green, it is tempting to say, "What did you do? You look like a friggin' leprechaun!" Rather than judging and demeaning her, we can deliberately focus on being curious. "Do you like the new color? What prompted you to dye your hair green? Is there anything I can do to help you with it?" We want her to know that we may not understand her intentions, but we respect her and value our relationship. We want her to feel seen and heard.

CONNECTION WITH GREATER HUMANITY

Astronauts have talked about seeing Earth from space and recognizing the oneness of human beings. Viewing Earth from this distance literally gave the astronauts a global perspective of humanity—we are one species that call this planet our home. This is known as the "Overview Effect." Divisions and disconnects are man-made, and they have been perpetuated over generations. Maybe we each need to make a pilgrimage to space to get a unifying, God's eye view of humanity.

Connection with humanity is the realization that humans all over the world have similarities. We tend to focus on the differences, which we now know is due to our negativity bias. We scan for differences because they could signify threats. Our negativity bias guides our brain to focus on possible danger, something different than what is familiar to us. Unfortunately, this blinds us to the potential beauty that could evolve from a new relationship.

Let's think about what we human beings have in common. Yes, we all have the basic physical needs for food and water, sleep, and safety. We also want to be healthy and loved. We want connections. We want what is best for our children. We have all experienced sadness, fear, confusion, and physical and mental pain. We have also experienced joy and happiness. Every human being has thoughts, ideas, feelings, and emotions. To feel connected to people of different races, in different countries, with a different language and culture, let's focus on our shared human experiences.

Connection leads to understanding and compassion. Compassion is a step deeper than connection. It means "to suffer with." The Dalai Lama described compassion through a story of a person getting crushed by a large rock. Compassion doesn't mean we get under the rock to feel what the other person is feeling. Compassion is doing what we can to remove the rock. (Gyatso, Tutu 2016, 259) What a powerful practice to suffer not only with people we know but also with people we've never met! Yet, we did it during the COVID-19 crisis. Health care providers practice compassion with strangers every day. We can choose to affect a piece of our shared world and the people within it.

HOW IS CONNECTION REFLECTED IN TRADITIONS?

A number of traditions teach that connection to ourself, one another, and spirit is important and comes from within. The practice of yoga emphasizes that awareness is already in us; we just have to awaken to it. It is a spiritual connection to ourself, the highest level of who we are. In connection with others, the Yoga Sutras recommend the discipline of speech. Only speak what is true, kind, and helpful. The sutras also highlight that no one can ever give us happiness or unhappiness; they can only reflect or distort our own inner happiness. It is like a mirror. What we perceive in others is partly based on what is happening inside of us. As we awaken to what's happening inside us, around us, and between us in our relationships, we have another opportunity to examine our mindset. This newly assessed mindset will likely grow our connections.

The teachings of Buddhism are deeply rooted in compassion. It advises that if we see the suffering in others, we should do what we can do to alleviate the suffering. This is service and purpose in action. It is also compassion. The Dali Lama says that when we see ourselves as separate from others, we create suffering within ourselves. If we think of others as different than us—different beliefs, different race, different economic status—we create walls to keep us apart from others. (Gyatso, Tutu 2016, 200) Compassion sees our sameness. Our common, innate humanness.

In the Jewish faith, relating to God is often done within a circle of community. Many of their practices, such as prayer, meals, study, and celebrations, involve a connection with people.

Christianity emphasizes a personal connection with the Holy Spirit—God dwells within each person. We are, therefore, in constant contact with God. This creates a continuous and undivided connection.

The Islamic prayer called Salat literally means "connection" in Arabic. It connects Muslims to Allah five times a day. Imam Abdul Malik Mujahid says that in Sharia, the Islamic way of life, it is only through serving human beings that they can connect to the Creator.

Faith communities—churches, synagogues, mosques—are connections among people who have similar beliefs. They create a significant feeling of belonging. These entities aim to offer shared experiences that deepen connections with other attendants as well as with the Divine. A core tenant of many religions is to help others, to connect with others. Because of the large group bond, faith communities often have more service impact than one or two individuals have.

Religion has had its challenges over thousands of years, actually severing connections between people. This is most often due to dogma, defined as "a fixed, especially religious, belief or set of beliefs that people are expected to accept without any doubts." (Cambridge Advanced Learners Dictionary 2021) Certain religions insist that their way is the only way to the Divine. This lends itself to judgment and anger, and the creation of a tribe versus the enemy—us versus them. Our authentic self and higher power are personal and about love. The Divine lives within each of us. If we give a stranger who is hungry something to eat or a stranger who is cold some extra clothing, we offer our love to the Divine—regardless of what the stranger calls their higher power. The Divine lives within them. The spirit within me salutes the spirit within you.

CHARACTER POWER TOOLS

Who do we get to become if we experience deep, true connection? Connection with our authentic self, with others, and with our higher power will deepen our awareness of our power tools. Our power tools can strengthen our practice of connection as well.

Courage

To effectively connect with ourselves, our higher power, and others, we have to expose ourselves. We need the courage to be vulnerable. If we go into hiding to prevent others from seeing all of us, our lives are a story that is only partly true. We use extra energy to keep that story going. This decreases the amount of available energy we have to do a deep dive into our connection work, within ourselves and with other people. To be vulnerable means, we risk getting hurt. Vulnerability is scary at first. Until we practice it. Then it becomes freeing. Vulnerability allows us to strip off our layers of protection—and some of us are wearing enough layers to survive in Antarctica—to discover our true self as well as true relationships.

Simplicity

Declutter those relationships that are merely distractions. The parents of your child's teammate who complain about everyone around them. Your wine club in which people only feel connected after drinking an ample supply of wine. Think about connections that are real and valuable to you. Spend your valuable time on them. And when you are with them, be with them. Don't use that time to scroll through social media. Social media connections are superficial relationships. People share fragments of information, information that is filtered and cultivated to look at a certain way. A deep, give-and-take conversation doesn't occur. We don't know people's full stories, only the chapters they selectively let us see. This doesn't represent a real connection.

Real connections are simple—we have our loved ones' backs, and they have ours. Our communications are clear and honest. When we give of ourselves to these relationships, we do so without expectations of praise or reciprocal treatment. We know we are mutually supportive of each other, no strings attached.

Positivity

We know that wishing our loved ones well, sending positive thoughts their way, or praying for them feels uplifting. It is a brief time of reflection and thankfulness for these dear connections. Have you ever sent someone you don't know positive thoughts? Doing so actually creates a feeling of connection between you and the stranger. Try it the next time you notice a jogger who is struggling during a hot day or a weary-looking mom pushing her children in a stroller. Use your method of choice—pray for them or silently wish them well.

Gossip and negative, judgmental comments are counter to our authentic self, connection to the Divine, and connections with others. Our authentic self is about love, truth, and peace. When we are connected to our authentic self and know what is going on inside us, we are less likely to talk badly to or about other people. Gossip is actually a method of connecting with others, although a lazy method. Our egoic self takes no issue with trying to feel good at the expense of other people. The brain releases the same excitatory chemicals as when we are exposed to negative media. Gossip can backfire and destroy relationships.

Consider checking in with yourself before communicating, especially in challenging conversations, by using the teachings of the yoga sutras:

1. Is it kind?

2. Is it helpful?

3. Is it true?

If what you are going to say doesn't meet these criteria, try finding another way to communicate it, or don't say it at all.

Commitment

The choice to stay connected to ourselves, our higher power, and others is just that—a choice. It is not a mandate. Choosing our connections on a regular basis allows us to consciously resolve that those relationships are our top priorities. Those are the relationships that are worth maintaining and strengthening.

One way to focus time and energy on our chosen connections is to reduce the number of mental inputs. Consider making a commitment to limit your time on social media. Create a balance that is healthy for you. Spend more time with your real, in-person connections. A number of studies show that reducing social media use improves our personal well-being. It also improves our relationships' well-being. How can we enhance our relationships with those who are sitting right next to us when we are interacting with Bjorn from Norway, the exchange student we barely knew in high school?

Let's commit to connecting with those that matter.

Resilience

A connection to others and to the Divine helps us become more resilient when we face challenges. We can lean on these valuable connections. How much easier is it to go to the gym when a friend is going with us? When we experience emotional struggles, a connection with a loved one or with the Divine provides reassurance and keeps us moving forward.

Maintaining and strengthening our connections requires resilience every day. In the face of distractions and disagreements, we can work on coming from a place of love to connect from an authentic level.

When we read about suffering or conflict in the news media, let's remember that negative news sells. We have to consciously resist experiencing a negative spiral from what we read in the media. To practice compassion and connection to people in the news, find a photo of a specific person. Think about what their life has been like? Look at their lives from different perspectives. When we connect a face to human suffering, we develop compassion and resist seeing the world as wholly negative.

Awareness

Our authentic self or inner voice has been with us all of the time. We simply need to uncover it, to become aware of it. Buddhist monk Haemin Sunim says that awareness is like looking for New York City when you are in New York City. You are already there. Awareness is available to us at all times; we just have to shut off distractions and tame our ping-pong-ball-like thoughts to find it.

Sometimes our connections feel uncomfortable and may trigger us in a certain way. What is the trigger? Why is the connection uncomfortable? These triggers are like bright yellow yield signs, telling us to slow down. To turn inward. Our next job is to uncover the layers of bias and self-judgment. What is our conditioned response, and is it still true to us? The triggers that pop up in our relationship with others lead to a greater awareness of ourselves.

We become aware of our authentic self through stillness, breath practice, and mindfulness. We become aware of how connections affect us by paying attention to how our body feels or responds.

Some of us connect to our higher power through emotionally intense experiences—music, nature, art, or witnessing something beautiful. It is a feeling like being lifted out of our body. Are you aware of such experiences that have taken your breath away? This can even include those moments when we look at our children and experience a sense of awe. It is a powerful sensation that there something bigger than us!

Purpose

When we are deeply connected to ourselves, it is possible to find our true purpose. We become aware of the unique way in which we can serve the world. Does something emotionally move you so much that you physically feel it in your body? These deep feelings are signals of your potential purpose. Some people think of this experience as "a calling." We feel called or pulled by our higher power to do the work. We want to show compassion—to suffer with—then work to alleviate the suffering. Our passionate service may directly affect others, like teaching or patient care. It may also affect nature and the environment, like keeping our rivers clean or repairing the ocean reefs. It is your purpose. You get to define it.

Purpose is the ultimate form of connection.

HOW CAN I APPLY CONNECTION TO MY PERSONAL LIFE?

- Once we check in with home base—ourselves—we are able to make deliberate decisions about who we want to connect with. Why do we want to connect with them? What is the best method to use to connect with them? To develop connection within ourselves, we need to take time to be silent, to be present. Set your alarm ten minutes earlier than usual so you have time to sit and breathe in the morning. Mornings work well to do this because our brain is still fresh. Our thoughts and activities of the day haven't had time to distract us yet. Remember, the more you practice, the stronger your relationship becomes and the more access you feel to your own guidance. Begin to notice the form your guidance comes in. It may present itself through hearing things, seeing images, noticing things, or being drawn to certain conversations or religious passages. It may also appear in your reaction to other people.

- Schedule time to feel awe. What takes your breath away? Music? Nature? Art?

- Take time to notice how good it feels to connect with others, to act with compassion.

HOW CAN CONNECTION HELP STRENGTHEN OUR MARRIAGE?

The Gottman Institute is renowned for its research on and study of marriage. They have studied couples for decades to examine the intricacies of marriage. Their website provides tools, resources, and quizzes to explore your marriage, repair your relationship, and build a deeper connection. It is available at www.gottman.com.

The strongest marriages have a deep sense of shared meaning. Sometimes the shared meaning is unspoken but mutually understood. An example of shared meaning is having a common set of values. Take some time with your partner to talk about your values. Why do you believe them? What do you want to do with them? Do you want to nurture them and act on them? Whatever you decide, you've consciously made the decision together, as a connected couple.

Listen until your partner feels heard. Do you ever have a conversation with your partner where you say, "Haven't we talked about this already?" or "Haven't we beaten this subject to death?" Connection thrives on feeling heard and understood, even if one person disagrees with the other. To actively listen:

1. Maintain eye contact. Yes, that means put down your electronic devices. Focus on what your partner is saying.

2. Ask questions to show that you are listening. "Wait, was Sally in the room with you when you tripped over the garbage can?"

3. Consider paraphrasing, such as, "So, you're saying that..."

4. Consider using empathizing comments, such as, "I bet you were so excited..."

- If you are looking for a specific response or action, ask for it. In clear terms. Don't assume your partner will read between the lines: "I am the only one who helps our son Hank with his math homework, and I do it every single day. It sure would be nice if someone else would take the time to help him." In this example, we didn't specifically ask our partner for their help. The following example provides a clearer ask, "Would you please help Hank with his math homework after dinner on Mondays and Wednesdays?" Another communication tool is to focus on what end result you both would like to see. "We both want Hank to understand and finish his math assignments. How can we work together to get to this result?"

- If your responses to your partner tend to be defensive and reactionary, especially when it comes to hot-button issues, try to pause and feel the defensiveness as it arises. This will take practice. After you pause, breathe, and visualize your defensiveness evaporating into thin air, your authentic self can choose a different response. We may need to take time during meditation to evaluate why those defensive feelings continue to arise. Getting into the habit of watching our feelings evolve and then dissolve before responding will give you more time and space for joy in your relationship.

- Think about how you and your partner most commonly connect. Are you more apt to connect emotionally, such as by discussing your feelings with each other about your day? Do you connect spiritually, such as meditating or praying together? Or, do you most commonly connect physically, such as through hugs, kisses, or sex? Highlight your strongest area of connection. Consider focusing on connecting with your partner in one of your lesser-practiced areas.

- Invest in quality time with your partner—time that you can focus solely on each other.

- Physically connect with your partner. Hugs, kisses, back rubs, sex, massages are physical ways to deepen connections between you and your partner. Also, consider different physical environments that foster connections:

- Calm, relaxing spaces. Create an inviting, cozy environment that oozes relaxation. This allows everyone to let go of the day's stress and feel at ease.

- Quiet spaces. Meditate or go to a yoga class together.

- Concerts, church, or your living room. Listen to music or sing together. Both activities increase oxytocin levels, one of the feel-good chemicals in our brain.

- Nature. Connect with each other in nature. Nature is closely linked with spirituality.

- Foodbanks, hospital, or a homeless shelter. Volunteer or do charity work together.

- A gym or workout facility. Do a workout while interacting with each other.

- Local colleges or universities. Take a class together, such as an Improv class or weekend course at a university.

- Events. Go to an event together—a theater production, an athletic event, an art show.

HOW CAN CONNECTION HELP STRENGTHEN OUR FAMILY RELATIONSHIP?

- Take care of the connections in your immediate family first. If things are "off" with any of your family connections, stand by for the impact it will have on other connections as well.

- Let your home become a safe home base, a place your children can always rely on. Be their strength, not another stressor.

- Take time to connect as a family regardless of how busy life gets. Get creative. Do a workout together as a family. Have breakfast together. Connect with each other during rides in the car. Just make sure you are focusing on each other, practicing your active listening.

- Demonstrate healthy connections for your children. Show them how powerful and meaningful bonds can be in a marriage and in a family.

- Think about each of your children's preferred love languages. Try showing them love in that way. Notice your child's response.

- Schedule date days and outings with each child, just the two of you—Mom and little Fred on one day and Dad and Fred on another day. One-on-one time deepens the bonds between a parent and child.

- Choose your words carefully. We can't erase what we say. How can we speak with the intention to connect rather than divide? When your children communicate, help them learn to focus on the questions, "Is it kind, is it true, and is it helpful?" If what they want to say does not meet those criteria, they can find another way to say it or not say anything at all.

- Take time for physical touch—hugs, fist bumps, high-fives, back rubs. These small bits of connection bond us more than we realize. We are wired for physical touch, and these interactions are becoming sparser due to our digital distractions. Keep in mind each child's preferred method of touch.

- Begin to teach your children how to connect with their intuition. Ask them what they notice in their body when they feel specific emotions—happy, worried, angry, or sad.

- Model kindness to help cultivate compassion in your children. Research suggests that compassion is contagious. Let's give the next generation a boost so they can carry it forward into their future.

SUMMARY

Connection is the feeling that we belong to someone or something. We feel safe. "[Deep] relationships are like emotional vitamins, sustaining us through tough times and nourishing us daily" (Goleman 2006).

Just be your whole, beautiful self. You will be amazed at the connections that bloom—ones that you will cherish because they are deeply rooted, healthy, and enduring.

CHAPTER 13

CONTENTMENT

Have you ever freaked out when something didn't go as planned? Maybe you hit a deer with your car, or your child was diagnosed with a health disorder. It is easy to want to scream, "This isn't fair!" or "Are you kidding me? Life shouldn't be this hard!" Unanticipated experiences occur every day. They don't even have to be momentous to derail our well-planned day, week, or life. Contentment eradicates freak-out episodes.

Contentment is acceptance for what is in the present moment, without expectations or an attachment to the end result. When we are content, we live life on its own terms rather than focus on how we think it should be. We appreciate what we have and where we are without using our energy wishing things were different. In some cultures, contentment is compared to enlightenment—the highest level of being.

Contentment is our deepest form of connection to ourselves. It's very hard to cultivate, though, without having built the other parts of our Self first—the construction we've been doing in the previous chapters. We need well-functioning layers of our Self to arrive at contentment. If we don't move our body and we eat like shit, our physical and mental bodies don't function as well. If we don't examine our mindset, we are more likely to blindly react to emotional content, and view that content as negative. Without discipline, we don't even know if we're on a path, so why show up and build a habit to the unknown? Without connection, we focus on our ego. We look to other people and things to fulfill us, and we view people who think differently than us as our adversaries. Contentment requires all other parts of our Self to be developed. Only then can we understand and accept the present state of our lives.

Contentment is a deep sense of trust and peace. We trust that where we are in the present moment is part of a bigger plan. We are like the blinking dot on a Google Maps App. The dot identifies our exact location on our path of life. We can see that we've come a long way, but the path ahead is blurred. We know we are going in the right direction, but we can't make out the specific paths. And our destination is simply off the map. We may or may not like where we are right now, but we have an underlying sense of peace during our journey. We know the path is leading us to the next correct turn. Our higher power comes into action here; not for control, but for connection, for reassurance when we don't understand where we are or what is going on.

Contentment is about how we relate to what is going on around us—not how we react to our emotions. When we relate to a situation, we base our thoughts and actions on reality. What are the hard facts of the situation? No interpretations, opinions, predictions, or assumptions are involved. For example, our partner calls to tell us they have to work late for the sixth night this week. We acknowledge the altered schedule without judging our partner. We feel angry and disappointed about the unexpected change in our plans, making a note to later talk about our joint schedule. We decide to postpone our kids' bedtimes and spend the evening with Grandma and Grandpa. We are choosing to act according to what's happening in reality. Notice we didn't assume anything about our partner, their priorities, our relationship, etc. Though we felt angry and disappointed, we didn't let those emotions interfere with what we said or did. Our evening was not ruined. We didn't react to our emotions. We related to the situation at hand, and we responded to the facts. We can be content and feel our emotions at the same time.

When we react to our emotions, we react to our interpretation of the situation. We base our thoughts and actions on our narrative. Our narrative is the story we quickly and creatively weave throughout the facts. It helps our brains make sense of the situation. But as we know, our narrative is only our perspective, and it can be wrong. It is based on our emotions, assumptions, predictions, and opinions. And on our ego. Our ego wants to protect us from feeling hurt, embarrassed, or out of control. In the partner-arriving-home-late scenario, reacting to our narrative turns our evening negative. We assume that our partner just wants to avoid the witching hour at home— the time of night around bedtime when we try to corral our tired, crabby kids. Either that, or maybe our partner's co-workers brought in some beer, and they are all sitting around drinking with their feet propped up on their desks. Now we're pissed! We react to our anger and disappointment by yelling at our partner and sulking the rest of the evening. Both our negativity bias and our attachment to the narrative are at work here. As we learned in the Mindset chapter, we need to consider the whole situation and assess the facts versus our narrative. Then we can consciously choose how we want to relate to the situation—respond to the facts that we can control or react to our emotions.

We are so busy in this phase of our lives. How on earth are we supposed to think about contentment? We've all had times when we felt impatient getting the kids ready for bed at night. When we finally finished the bedtime routine, we slumped down in our favorite chair. We were so exhausted that we couldn't form words to discuss what we did during the day. Our fast-paced life is part of the reason to talk about this subject. Some days during this part of our journey, especially with children, seem to go on forever. We are physically and mentally busy. We don't often get to appreciate the immediate results of our profound parenting skills. The days may be long, but the years go by in a heartbeat. We then wish we had spent more time simply enjoying moments with our young family. In the life of a parent, practicing contentment can help our days feel more purposeful and fulfilling. We learn to appreciate the little changes in our children and their small victories during their growing years. And we learn to be at peace during the process, even amid the commotion that happens all around us. Contentment can coexist with busyness and discomfort.

When we are content, we detach ourselves from the reward or final result. We can work hard and do our best to make the result possible, but we can't control the result itself. Factors other than us contribute to the result. In other words, the journey belongs to us; the reward is out of our hands. We can control our efforts. Contentment doesn't depend on reaching some milestone or result. When it comes to parenting, what is the final result anyway? Is it tangible? Is it even under our control? "I'll know that I have been a good parent if my child gets into a D1 college and makes the basketball team as a freshman." What if that doesn't happen? We didn't achieve the result we wanted, so did we fail as a parent? Did our child fail us?

Or we could choose to be present in the little moments that make up a childhood. We can control our emotions and our efforts during our children's short journey with us—we cannot control the results.

CONTENTMENT IS NOT...

Contentment does not mean we are settling or being complacent. Contentment means we accept our situation or state of being as it is. We act with a clear mind. We accept the reality of now, and we are grateful for how far we have come. This doesn't detract us from our growth trajectory or improving what we have. Contentment doesn't hold us back. In fact, it allows us to move forward with a calm, alert brain.

Discontentment causes us to wallow in our distress, to feel hopeless. As we've learned, our brain doesn't work as well when we are distressed. Our brainpower is limited because it is focused on how unfair our situation is. Ultimately, discontentment is immobilizing. It stifles our growth.

Contentment is not based on productivity or contingencies. Many of us grew up thinking that if we weren't busy, working hard, or fretting, we weren't pulling our weight. We were lazy. We tied our productivity to our worthiness. We are all worthy. Period. Realizing our inherent worthiness is a predecessor to knowing contentment. Contentment is about being present during our daily actions, not attaching our sense of worth to them or to anything outside of ourselves. To develop contentment, we must disconnect our worthiness and self-love from our goals and results. "When I lose twenty pounds, I'll look good in a swimming suit. Then I'll feel happy and want to go to the public pool." This may be true, but as we know, happiness is a transient feeling. Once we achieve the twenty-pound weight loss, we will be happy until what—until we realize we have bat wings hanging under our arms? Now we decide we won't be happy until we fill our saggy arm skin with rock-hard muscles. Then what? The nice thing about contentment is that we can love ourselves right now, in the moment, while still working on our bat wings. It is healthy to have goals; it is not healthy to attach our well-being to those goals.

Contentment is not the same as happiness. The concept of happiness has been a hot-button issue for the last decade. It seems like the internet and bookstores are full of material about happiness—how and where to find it, how to keep it, how to share it with others. Yet it is different than contentment? The two concepts are different, though not mutually exclusive. Happiness is an emotion. Contentment is a state of being. Happiness is a reaction from sources outside of ourselves. It is an emotion that ebbs and flows. If we get a surprise bonus of $5000 at the end of the year, we feel happy. It is an emotional reaction to an outside source. Two months later, we've spent the $5000 on an old, used car, and we don't feel as happy; we are back to baseline. Contentment is a decision rather than a reaction. We can be content while we are happy that we received the bonus. We can still be content two months later after we've spent the money and the elation is gone. Contentment is a state of being that only comes from within us. It gives us power and stability, so we don't have to be swayed by our emotions.

Cole talks about many years of discontent that shaped her feelings and actions. She fought against reality during that time. She did not win. After her car accident, she longed to be back in her athletic, pain-free body. As she continued to fight against the reality of her injured body, her pain only grew worse. Once she became aware that she was engaged in a losing battle, she accepted her reality. I have injuries. This is my current situation. My body needs care and time to heal. I will begin to train it with love and acceptance. She loves the body she lives in today and continues to train it daily. It is strong and can stand up to the rigors of this reality.

Cole and her husband married when her husband was still immersed in medical school. They frequently moved to different locations during his years of medical training. Never quite feeling settled, doing her best to raise three young children, and taking out loans to pay rent, Cole dreamed of a stable life—to establish a home and lay down roots. Thinking back to this era, Cole laments the moments that she wished away. She feels she missed opportunities to have more good days, more meaningful connections, and more peaceful interactions. She wasn't yet living mindfully, not fully content. Thankfully, she didn't miss it all. Her husband completed his training, and the family moved to their current location as owners of their first home.

Cole felt like she went from being a single mom who barely lived paycheck-to-paycheck to being a "doctor's wife" within a day. She realized that a story had already been written about her by unknown authors, featuring her as the main character—a doctor's wife, a stay-at-home mom, a woman who enjoys frequent lunches out with friends, a woman who lounges by the pool at the local country club, and a woman who has no aspirations of her own. But this story belonged to others, not to Cole. She didn't author it, and she didn't turn over her naming rights to be featured in this story. Introductions in the community would begin, "This is Dr. B's wife." Um, she thought, my name is Nicole, and the story of what it means to be his wife is yours, not mine. Stories continue now that all of her children are in school. She gets asked if she can find enough work to do to fill her days. All she responds is, "Yes." To herself, she thinks I teach and coach adults, I own a company, I teach yoga, and I'm writing a book! Yet, she knows that she is the author of her own story. She doesn't need to be attached to the opinions of others—it is a deep feeling of contentment to live what is true for ourselves.

Jake talks about spending most of his young adult life chasing money and material things that had little true meaning to him. He thought that in order to feel content, he needed to graduate from college, get a job, work his way up the corporate ladder, buy a large house while building a hefty 401K, then buy a cottage—oh, and a boat. Yet, as he checked things off that list, he felt empty, like he would never "arrive." He didn't know how to be present in his day-to-day life because he was always focused on the final result. He put his nose to the grindstone and refused to feel happy until he accomplished his goal. But even when he did hit his goal, the happiness faded. Today, during his morning meditation, Jake prays that God will perform a small miracle and instill contentment in him. He wants to enjoy the little moments on his path. He doesn't want to always be looking for the next big thing, the next high.

HOW DO WE PERSONALLY DEVELOP CONTENTMENT?

Create space

We need to make space in our minds, hearts, and lives to be able to experience true contentment. We make space through silence, breath practice, and mindfulness. Mindfulness is one of the most studied practices for calming our body and mind—focusing on the present moment without judging. Prayer can be a form of mindfulness. We can release our thoughts and emotions and hand them to our higher power during our time of prayer. Meditation is another practice used to make space in the mind. With meditation, we focus our minds on a specific thought, object, sound, or pattern. Regardless of which tool we use to make space in our minds, it is important to practice it daily. We don't need to practice it for hours like we're living in a monastery. We are regular humans with busy lives! We can start with three minutes per day. What's most important is doing something that has meaning to you. Daily practice is like cleaning our eyeglasses each morning. We wipe away yesterday's smudges. We then look within ourselves as well as the outside world with new, clear lenses. If we don't clear our minds regularly, our lenses become increasingly cloudy. We begin to lose sight of our inner self and how it relates to others. Thankfully, we can clean our dirty lenses. We just need to make space and time to do so.

Get rid of the emotional suitcase

Many of us carry our emotions around with us like an old, battered suitcase. Yes, we need to wholly feel our emotions, but we do not need to collect and store them. When we think such thoughts or emotions like "I am happy, I am not very smart, and I am an angry person," we hold onto them. We add them to our suitcase. But these are thoughts and emotions—we feel happy, we think that we aren't smart, and we feel angry. Thoughts and emotions are fluid; they are fleeting. They don't define us. We are bigger, more expansive, and contain an underlying peace that stabilizes us. We are the only ones responsible for storing our emotions. We ultimately choose the weight of our baggage.

To clarify, emotions are healthy. Holding onto our emotions is unhealthy. Emotions are signals we use to alert and guide us. We can identify them, thank them for appearing, learn from them, then let them go. This is contentment. And contentment remains steady while our emotions ebb and flow. Let's decide to lighten our emotional suitcase. It drags us down and slows our progression on our journey.

Practice gratitude

Gratitude practice has been an integral exercise in developing many parts of our Self. We know what gratitude is. How do we practice it to develop contentment? Contentment is about the present moment. So, let's look around us and within us. What are we grateful for in the moment? Are we grateful for our current surroundings? For the storm clouds that are building near the horizon? For the opportunity to sit at our child's game and watch them enjoy their sport? For the smells coming from the grill as we prepare a meal? Sometimes, we complicate gratitude practice by searching for more grandiose things. When we appreciate little things, such as watching a long line of ants march single-file into their hole, we experience the simplicity of contentment. We can practice gratitude when we make space in our minds. We focus on our breath and on one thing for which we are grateful. Prayer can come into action here as well. One feature of prayer includes thanksgiving—it helps cultivate an awareness of our higher power's presence and availability in each moment.

Set limits for ourselves and simplify

We know that simplifying our life helps us focus on what is most meaningful to us. It removes the physical and mental clutter so that we more clearly see the present moment. And be content. Then why, when we feel uncomfortable or feel like something is "off," do we react by acquiring new stuff and adding more to our plates? More stuff and more action create excitement but also distraction. Until they aren't fresh and new anymore. It is a never-ending cycle. Our society says we shouldn't feel uncomfortable, so we should do whatever we can to avoid feeling it. This is where we set our limits—we will feel and work through our discomfort without adding anything more to our lives. We will learn from the discomfort. What will we decide to do with it? Will we act on its guidance, then let it go? Or will we hold onto it and haul it around in our emotional suitcase? Do we want heavier baggage? We can choose another way.

Work toward goals without fixating on the results

We are in control of our efforts toward a goal. We can do everything in our power and dedicate our efforts to a result. Our work and commitment to the goal are already making a difference. It is like relentlessly practicing our basketball skills for six months. We are in charge of our efforts. Our goal is to make the varsity team. However, we know that other factors will affect our ultimate goal. The results of such goals are beyond our control. Other players are vying for the same goal. We can't control the other players. The coaches are evaluating each of the players. We can't control the coaches. When we fixate only on the end result like it is a do-or-die situation, we hang our contentment on something outside of ourselves—something that is beyond our control. Our serious effort and practice may not get us our goal, the result we think we should get. If we don't achieve our "should" goal, making the varsity team, was our effort and practice a waste of six months? Did we not learn anything during that time? We certainly learned some life skills—discipline, courage, commitment, and resilience. We also vastly improved our basketball skills and learned some new moves. We can't erase a part of our life because we didn't achieve our chosen end result. We would erase part of our growth. Results were happening all along, but we weren't present to appreciate them.

Celebrate small milestones

In the above scenario, what small milestones could we have celebrated? The first time we landed five free throws in a row? When we played a game of one-on-one with our sports idol? When we increased our stamina and endurance from ten minutes to fifty minutes? Celebrating small milestones is a form of gratitude. It reminds us to be content during the process—the process of practicing, working, learning, and growing.

Give to others without expecting anything in return

Contentment leads to generosity. When we give to others with a generous heart, our brain releases positive, feel-good endorphins. Brain scans have shown that when we show compassion to others, the same reward centers light up as when we think of chocolate! The brain also releases oxytocin, the chemical that fosters connection and bonding—as well as reducing inflammation in our heart and blood vessels. Giving to others is mentally, physically, and spiritually healthy!

HOW DO WE DEVELOP CONTENTMENT IN OUR MARRIAGE?

We don't often associate "marriage" with the word "contentment." They simply aren't common word associations in our society. Discontentment in marriages is the reason marriage counselors are in such high demand. Discontentment occurs when one or both partners doesn't feel satisfied. They may feel unhappy and resentful. Often, one partner relies on the other for their own fulfillment—which we know isn't healthy and can't be sustained. Our society is oriented toward achieving the next big thing and making sure it feels good. But the lusty, feel-good feelings don't linger forever. Again, fulfillment needs to come from within us. Contentment can follow as we accept our marriage in the present moment with a peaceful heart.

When we are personally content, we accept our partner for who they are—rather than how we'd like them to be. (This does not apply to unhealthy or abusive behavior.) We remove phrases, such as,

"I wish he'd get his head out of the clouds and stop living in the future."

"I wish he'd dress better. The ripped sweatshirt he wears is still from high school!"

"I wish she was more outgoing and liked to spend time with people as much as I do."

Many of these wishes or expectations come from our mindsets. Is it time to examine more of those subconscious beliefs? We love our partner, but don't always like their actions. Though we have disagreements and annoyances, we are committed to working through them. We can do this respectfully because of our underlying state of contentment. We know we are journeying through this life together, sometimes on a different path, but going in the same direction. Let's try to encourage our partner and focus on what we appreciate about them.

Love doesn't have expectations or contingencies. We can control what we ask of our partner and in what manner we ask for it. We can ask our partner not to wear his ripped sweatshirt. Now it is out of our control. Our partner's choice is within his control. He responds, "I love you, and please don't take my decision personally. I want to wear my ripped sweatshirt because it is comfortable. More importantly, it is the last thing my dad bought for me." If our partner doesn't want to do something we request, it is because they don't want to do it. We don't need to read any more into it. We don't have to take it personally or create a narrative about how they arrived at their decision. We don't need to base our happiness or contentment on their choice. Thankfully, we know that our contentment comes from within us.

As the years pass in marriages, we often witness two separate identities merge into one. We see this when one partner speaks for the other, corrects the other's mistakes, or controls the other's actions. Let's remember that a marriage relationship is one whole that consists of two halves. We are responsible for our half only. If we try to control the other half, the relationship is based on fear and goes to hell. (Ruiz, Mills 1999, 66) Love has no obligations. It is content. Fear is full of obligations. It is far from content.

When we are individually content, we are able to give of ourselves without expecting anything in return. This doesn't have to include physical gifts. It can be about doing little things for each other. We can surprise our partner by getting their car washed, going to their favorite restaurant, or saying, "I love you. I'm so grateful that I met you!"

In content marriages, it is completely normal to experience a wide range of emotions with our partner. We can be grateful for our marriage while feeling difficult emotions. This is particularly reassuring during those rare times when we feel annoyed with our partner, like when they snore. In this case, we accept the facts of the situation: our partner is lying flat on their back and snoring. Loudly. We maintain an underlying sense of peace and contentment while we gently push them out of bed, feigning surprise when they wake up on the floor. Contentment involves a little humor as well.

HOW DO WE DEVELOP CONTENTMENT AS A FAMILY?

The American dream conditions us to want. It's deeply ingrained in us at a young age. We want the colorful cereal with the character on the box, the sparkly dress, the newest phone, the latest video game. We want our kids to look and act a certain way. Some of us want our kids to be more—be more responsible, be more athletic, be more musical, or be more academic. Do you think today's society teaches children contentment? Are there ever enough youth activities, sports, and associated camps? It seems that some people keep an invisible curriculum vitae for each of their children—a CV that starts soon after birth. The more activities our children participate in, the more awards they receive, and the more fulfilled they become. Is this what we want for them? Do we want to teach them to feel fulfilled from external sources?

Boredom is a foreign concept to many of our children. It is uncomfortable. Society has written a script for young people today, "More toys, more stuff, more activities—I need other people, activities, and things to prevent me from becoming bored." An unfortunate result of the constant desire for more and better is that our kids are physically paying for it. Discontent is stressful. Some symptoms of stress in children include stomachaches, headaches, or moodiness. When we provide space for boredom, the brain has an opportunity to search for interest, passion, connection, and recovery.

Think about social media and contentment, or should we say discontentment? With social media, we watch other people's highlight reels. Recall that highlight reels are the best short clips from a movie that end up on the promotional trailer. When we compare the highlight reels of others to the entirety of our own lives, outtakes and all, we don't feel like we match up. It is nearly impossible to be content while monitoring social media unless we are aware of the behind-the-scenes illusions.

Have you ever gone to dinner at a restaurant and noticed an entire family glued to their phones or similar devices? Nobody is experiencing the present moment or in connection with anyone at the table. Where is the contentment? If contentment is about the present moment, smart devices take us away from the present moment. And away from each other. How can we practice contentment and connection with each other when our minds are enjoying time in cyberspace? We are well aware that going to a restaurant as a family gives us numerous opportunities to feel uncomfortable. We also know that being fully present together as a family is valuable. What do we do? We start with one small action. We can take a small step toward being present with our family. This may include having one meal together without smart devices. It may include playing a board game together. It may even include spending two minutes together to watch the sunset. Continue to add small steps, even if they are baby steps.

HOW IS CONTENTMENT REFLECTED IN TRADITIONS?

Contentment is like a thread that weaves through all traditions and religions. It is a sense of wholeness.

In yoga, attachments are forms of energy. Energy is meant to flow through us, not get stuck in our body. Yoga focuses on non-attachment to material things, the outcomes of actions, thoughts, and feelings. The yogic belief is that trapped energy—including emotions—can lead to pain, suffering, and disease. Non-attachment allows us to define ourselves authentically and to experience connections on a deeper level. Letting go of attachments and thinking of them as energy can bring us peace.

Buddhism has a similar concept to that of yoga. Simply said, Buddhism considers contentment the ultimate wealth. "Health is the greatest gift. Contentment is the greatest wealth." Buddhism also emphasizes balance in our lives— contentment is a part of a balanced life. "Life is about balance. Be kind, but don't let people abuse you. Trust, but don't get deceived. Be content, but never stop improving yourself."

A Hasidic proverb states, "While we pursue happiness, we flee from contentment." We aren't mindful of the present.

Islam teaches us to be content with what Allah has given us, and we will be among the richest people. Wealth, children, house, and talents—be content with your share of these things.

Throughout the Christian Bible, people are called to keep their eyes on God, to trust in Him, and to know that He will provide. Philippians 4:12-13 says, "I know what it is to be in need, and I know what it is to have plenty. I have learned the secret of being content in any and every situation, whether well-fed or hungry, whether living in plenty or in want. I can do all things through Him who gives me strength." Hebrews 13:5 says, "Keep your life free from the love of money, and be content with what you have, for He has said, 'I will never leave you or forsake you.'"

CHARACTER POWER TOOLS

Who do we get to become if we experience contentment? Our power tools will help us develop and practice contentment. Being content will also help us further develop our power tools.

Courage

To practice being content in our day-to-day activities, we have to let go of our deep attachment to the result. We live in a results-oriented society. As we said, it is useful to have goals. It is not healthy to attach our happiness to the outcomes of those goals. This may go against some of our instinctual mindsets, such as Put your head down, work long hours, and don't come up for breath until that project is complete. This may have worked for Bill Gates, but it's not a healthy option for most people. We spend most of our lives in the "in-between"—the area between setting a goal and getting the result. Since we have a lot of living left to do, why don't we try to be content in the in-between? We need to continually reassure ourselves that we are okay right where we are today, in the present moment.

It takes courage to be content during a struggle, to be joyful and uncomfortable at the same time. We know that life is full of change, fraught with highs and lows. Knowing that we are on the right path and taking baby steps forward, we don't need to freak out when we don't feel in control.

Simplicity

Contentment is simple, but we don't realize it. We are distracted by external inputs, material possessions, other people, and our own mental clutter. We need to understand that we are our own source of contentment. That is the ultimate simplicity. Detaching from material things and external inputs provides clarity and fosters contentment.

Positivity

To cultivate contentment, look for the good and be the good in situations—without ties to a reward. It takes the ego out of the equation. Contentment is our internal therapist telling us that we can stand right where we are with gratitude and a peaceful heart.

On the other hand, negativity breeds discontentment. Discontentment is like arguing with reality—we will not accept "what is" in the present moment. "What is" should change. This is really a no-win situation. The present moment is what it is. Now, what do we want to do with it?

Commitment

Life is full of surprises—and surprises come in many forms. We may experience an unexpected victory, a devastating loss, or simply be thrown so far off our path that we land in a distant cornfield. Being content in our missteps and challenges takes a practice of commitment. Contentment doesn't see mistakes as failing; it sees them as learning. If we don't crash and burn during our journey, we can't be after something very big. Mistakes will happen. Let's accept that. We can commit to the work, know our goals, and hop back on the path. If we don't learn and fail along the way, we don't grow. If we aren't growing, we are slowly dying.

Awareness

Since we have opted for a path of growth, we routinely push ourselves toward goals. This is fine as long as we don't attach our experience of contentment to these goals. This will take awareness. We need to celebrate our efforts and our progress toward the goals. We don't need the reward, attention, or accolades.

Awareness also allows us to choose our reaction to our present reality. We can choose to look at it negatively and fight it. Or we can choose to accept it and move forward with a clear mind.

Taming our ego will help us become content. Recall that our ego controls our should and shouldn't thoughts. It's hard to be content in the present moment when our ego screams, "I can't accept this reality because I should have won the race, I should have been put on the varsity team, I shouldn't have to suffer like I am." Our true self is positive, humble, and giving. Our ego wants the outside world to make us happy. It says, "If it feels good, I'll keep going. If it starts to hurt, I'm done." Our ego is always searching for the next big thing; it is never satisfied for long. How does that coincide with contentment? Contentment is not the ego. Contentment comes from within us—only from our authentic self.

Resilience

It is challenging to be content when we feel uncomfortable. Our ego naturally wants to blame someone or safely hide in a pocket of comfort or sameness. The more that we associate contentment with inner peace, the more resilient we become to discomfort. This will take conscious practice. Since contentment enhances our inner strength and reduces overall stress, we are more equipped to handle challenges. Regardless of what is going on outside of us, we can accept where we are in the present moment.

Contentment is a way of being that essentially makes us resilient to the stressors of life.

Purpose

Living with purpose is making conscious choices in our day-to-day life that honor our values, passions, unique talents, and gifts. In essence, we choose to live life on purpose. Earlier in the book, we referred to our choices as dots in a complicated dot-to-dot puzzle. We have days in which we feel we are simply moving from one dot to another—the connection doesn't create a clear picture. We accept where we are during those days. We are content and continue to do the work of refining our Self. Until suddenly, we catch a glimpse of something beautiful, a work of art that looks like a masterpiece in the making. That beautiful work of art is our purpose in action.

When we give of ourselves according to our purpose, we offer a portion of our art. We can't control whether or not the recipient will accept our gift. The outcome does not belong to us. We serve without any attachment to a reward or acknowledgment. This is true contentment. The more we practice kindness without expecting rewards, the more content we become.

HOW CAN I APPLY CONTENTMENT PERSONALLY?

To experience contentment, we need to practice creating space on a regular basis using our tools of breath work and mindfulness. Where will that fall in your daily schedule?

When can you find time to explore questions like these?

- Have you attached emotions, such as happiness or satisfaction, to some type of outcome? If so, can you control the outcome? How can you alter your thinking patterns so that you focus on and be content with the process?

- Listen for the stories of what you are supposed to do or be. Is that true to you, or is that someone else's story?

- Are you fighting with reality? In what ways could you accept what is real in the present moment?

- Do you have a deity, symbol, or principle that is meaningful to you? If so, how can you use that consistently?

- What do you know for sure that you are on earth to do? This can be something small and tangible or grandiose and ethereal. What is the next step to move closer to that purpose?

- When are you at peace? What helps you experience that peace?

- How and where can you eliminate comparing yourself to others? We can never be content when we try to be someone else.

HOW CAN CONTENTMENT STRENGTHEN OUR MARRIAGE?

- What are you grateful for in your partner? What are you grateful for in your partnership, your marriage?

- Think about times that you feel annoyed with your partner. Is there a story associated with these times that your partner may not even be aware of? How can you cultivate acceptance and empathy toward your partner?

- Embrace the process of growth as individuals and as a partnership. Support and encourage each other.

- Remember that you can be content in your marriage while experiencing emotions. Just don't hang onto those emotions.

- Discuss what is enough with each other. How will you model this?

- Discuss how contentment in your marriage will help foster contentment as parents.

HOW CAN CONTENTMENT STRENGTHEN OUR FAMILY RELATIONSHIP?

We model contentment for our children. They see what we do and want to do the same thing. How can we demonstrate contentment? We can practice gratitude with them. We can reduce our impulse buys and the amount of stuff we bring into the house.

- How can you experience presence with your family? Do you have set times that are device-free? Do you have scheduled times that you can focus on each other without distractions?

- Consider having limits on stuff and organized activities. More is definitely not always better.

- Consider your child's choice of activities, especially organized ones. How can you constructively encourage and support your child without tying your emotions to their performance?

- Be aware of signs of stress in your children— stomachaches, headaches, moodiness, new fears, teeth grinding or clenching, or simply not wanting to leave your side.

- Practice doing nice things without expecting a reward or acknowledgment. Write a nice note or give an anonymous gift to a friend or stranger.

- Find joy in giving away what "belongs" to you. Clean out closets, go through Christmas decorations, whatever you hang onto because you've always had it around the house. Practice detachment together, especially related to material things.

SUMMARY:

In some cultures, contentment is one of the highest levels of spiritual achievement, somewhat like enlightenment. We are unconditionally whole regardless of what's happening around us. We are simply revealing our wholeness to ourselves layer by layer. Contentment takes practice, but we can achieve it. It is so worth it! Many practices foster our experience of contentment. We can make space for breath work and mindfulness, practice gratitude, learn to let our emotions flow through us, refuse to let our contentment be contingent on results, celebrate small milestones, and give to others without expectations. We need to practice being fully present during the growth process of life. It is a practice of being and becoming at the same time.

Even though our days are full and our to-do list is long, contentment is a constant inner peace. We accept what is in the present moment. It provides an underlying steadiness during this journey of life. A beautiful reality is that our journey—the building of our Self, our path of mastery—has no endpoint. We will never cross a finish line. We get to grow continuously until the end of our days on this earth. At age 115.

If we are going to be around that long, wouldn't we rather be content along the way?

GOING FORWARD

In order to create a peaceful family, we must first create inner peace and joyfulness in our self. Then we can share it with our family. They can share it with others. Peace can spread from one family to ten families to hundreds of families. That way, we can change and bring a happier community, happier society, then happier humanity (Gyatso, Tutu 2016, 295). We must build our Self first; then we can share our love, joy, and peace with our family.

We equated building our Self to building a home, a home that will always be undergoing improvements. And we can be content with that. Our home requires daily maintenance for optimal performance. Keep in mind that each person in our family has their own home to build—their own individual Self. As a family unit, though, our homes are interconnected. All family members get to maintain this greater structure as well as their individual Self. Does this sound like a lot of work? With a healthy body, a strong mind, and a peaceful spirit, we can do it. It's time to own your home—only you can do that. So, grab your power tools, and let's keep building!

REFERENCES

Basso, Julia C. and Suzuki, Wendy A. 2017. "The Effects of Acute Exercise on Mood, Cognition, Neurophysiology, and Neurochemical Pathways: A Review." Brain Plasticity 2, no. 2: 127-152.

Battle, Roxane. 2017. *Pockets of Joy: Deciding to Be Happy, Choosing to be Free.* New Kensington, PA: Whitaker House.

Becker, Josh. 2018. *The More of Less: Finding the Life you Want Under Everything You Own.* Colorado Springs, CO: Water Brook.

Breast Cancer.org. 2020. "Nutrition and Breast Cancer Risk Reduction." Last modified November 18, 2020. https://www.breastcancer.org/tips/nutrition/reduce_risk.

Brito, Leonardo B., Djalma R. Ricardo, Denise Sardinha Mendes Soares de Araujo, Plinio Santos Ramos, Jonathon Myers, and Claudio Gil Soares de Araujo. 2014. "Ability to sit and rise from the floor as a predictor of all-cause mortality." European Journal of Preventive Cardiology 21, no.7: 892-898.

Brown, Brene. 2015. *Rising Strong.* New York: Penguin Random House.

Buettner, Dan. 2012. *The Blue Zones, second Edition: 9 Lessons for Living Longer from the People Who've Lived the Longest.* Washington D.C.: National Geographic.

Cambridge Advanced Learner's Dictionary. May 5, 2021. http://www.dictionary.cambridge.org/us/dictionary/english/dogma.

Chen, Ying, Eric S. Kim, Howard K. Koh, Lindsay A. Frazier, and Tyler J. VanderWeele. 2019. "Sense of mission and subsequent health and well-being among young adults: An outcome-wide analysis." American Journal of Epidemiology 188, no. 4: 664-673.

Dalai Lama [Tenzin Gyatso] and Desmond Tutu. 2016. The Book of Joy: Lasting Happiness in a Changing World. With Douglas Abrams. New York: Avery.

Damon, William. 2009. *The Path to Purpose: How Young People Find Their Calling in Life.* New York: Free Press.

Divine, Mark. 2015. *Unbeatable Mind* 3rd ed. Printed by the author.

Divine, Mark. 2020. *Staring Down the Wolf.* New York: St. Martin's Press.

Ferguson, Michael et al. 2018. "Reward, salience, and attentional networks are activated by religious experience in devout Mormans." Social Neuroscience 13, no. 1:104-116

Frankl, Viktor. 2014. *Man's Search for Meaning.* Revised ed. Boston, MA: Beacon Press.

Gerritsen, Roderik J.S. and Guido P.H. Band. 2018. "Breath of Life: The Respiratory Vagal Stimulation Model of Contemplative Activity." Frontiers in Human Neuroscience 12, no. 397:9.

Goleman, Daniel. 2006 *Social Intelligence: The New Science of Human Relationships*. New York: Bantom Books.

Graziano Breunig, Loretta. 2016. *Habits of a Happy Brain*. Avon, MA: Adams Media.

Hanson, Rick. 2013. *Hardwiring Happiness: The New Brain Science of Contentment, Calm, and Confidence*. New York: Harmony.

Hawkins, David. 2012. *Power vs. Force: The Human Determinants of Human Behavior*. USA: Hayhouse.

Lakerfield, Jeroen, Anne Loyen, Nina Schotman, Carel F. W. Peeters, Greet Cardon, Hidde P van der Ploeg, Nanna Lien, Sebastien Chastin, and Johannes Brug. 2017. "Sitting Too Much: A hierarchy of socio-demographic correlates." Preventative Medicine 101:77.

Loehr, Jim and Schwartz, Tony. 2003. *The Power of Full Engagement*. New York: The Free Press.

Mann, Sandi. 2016. *The Science of Boredom: Why Boredom is Good*. London: Robinson.

Maslow, Abraham H. 1970. *Motivation and Personality*. New York: Harper & Row.

McGinnis, Scott. 2021. "Exercise can boost your memory and thinking skills." Harvard Health Publishing. February 15, 2021. http://www.health.harvard.edu/mind-and-mood/exercise-can-boost-your-memory-and-thinking-skills.

Merriam-Webster.com Dictionary, s.v. "Vulnerability," accessed April 3, 2021, https://www.merriam-webster.com/definition/vulnerability.

Ruiz, Don Miguel and Janet Mills. 1999. *The Mastery of Love*. San Rafael, CA: Amber-Allen.

Satter, Ellyn. "Raise a Healthy Child who is a Joy to Feed." Ellyn Satter Institute. 2019. http://www.ellynsatterinstitute.org/how-to-feed/the-division-of-responsibility-in-feeding/.

"Selecting Nutrient-dense Food for Good Health." Journal of the Academy of Nutrition and Dietetics. 2016. http://eatrightpro.org/practice-paper-nutrient-density.

Smolak, L. 2011. *Body Image: A Handbook of Science, Practice, and Prevention*. 2nd ed. New York: Guilford.

Suzuki, Wendy. "The brain-changing benefits of exercise." TED: Ideas Worth Spreading, March 21, 2018, https://www.ted.com/talks/wendy_suzuki_the_brain_changing_benefits_of_exercise.

Ward, Robert. 2016. "The True Meaning of Parental Commitments". Rewarding Education. October 5, 2016. http://www.rewardingeducation.wordpress.com/2016/10/5/the-true-meaning-of-parental-commitments/.

Vaish, Amrisha, Tobias Grossman, Amanda Woodward. 2008. "Not all emotions are created equal: The negativity bias in social-emotional development." Psychological Bulletin 134, no. 3: 383-403.

Walker, Matthew. 2018. *Why we Sleep: Unlocking the Power of Sleep and Dreams.* New York: Scribner.

ACKNOWLEDGMENTS

As siblings, we have deep and eternal appreciation for our parents who raised us with constant love and support. We have been well-loved and encouraged from not only our parents but both sets of grandparents, who have each been married for sixty-five plus years. We are grateful to our extended family and the families we have been fortunate enough to marry into. It has been the gift of a life-time. Thank you to each and every one of you.

To our spouses and children who give our lives meaning. We are grateful for your love, support, and willingness to do the work right alongside of us.

We are forever grateful to Robin Elvig without whom this book would not exist. Her ability to make our vision a reality came with remarkable tenacity, love, and wit. Thank you, Robin, from the bottom of our hearts.

Thank you to Amber Vilhauer, Amber Kidd, Lauden Davis, Megan O'Malley, Ekaterina Nikitina, Sharon Ludwig, Brandon Priebe, Manny Leon and the entire team at NGNG Enterprises who supported every step of launching this book out into the world. We couldn't have done it without you!

Thank you to Ashley Bunting at Merack Publishing who patiently supported us through the publishing process.

To the Total Potential community of badass moms and dads who are courageous enough to love deeply, grow daily, and create the family life of their dreams. We do this every day for you.

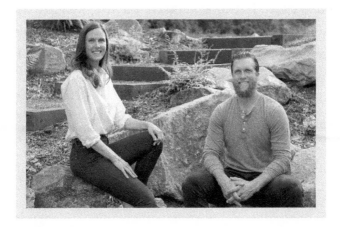

ABOUT THE AUTHORS

Cole Berschback and Jake Taylor are siblings and co-founders of Total Potential.

Cole has trained extensively in the health and wellness field to work as an Unbeatable Mind Coach, Registered Dietitian, and RYT 200 Certified Yoga Instructor. She loves supporting deep and meaningful transformation of others. Her greatest joy is experiencing life with her husband and three children. She has a long sustaining faith that guides her toward purpose-driven work.

Jake Taylor is anchored to a deep Christian faith. He loves growing alongside his wife and supporting his children in carving their own path and chasing their dreams with relentless effort. Jake loves CrossFit, Jiu Jitsu, hunting, fishing and all things outdoors. He spent seven years in the American Hockey League before retiring from professional sports. He is a CrossFit Level 1 Trainer and Unbeatable Mind Coach.

ABOUT THE AUTHORS